"WHAT'S GOING ON IN THERE?"

The Anatomy of a Resistance Training Set

THE NEUROMUSCULAR SYSTEM • CHEMICAL INTERACTIONS
ENERGY SYSTEMS & FATIGUE • GENETIC INFLUENCES
SKILL & TRAINING • MOTIVATION FACTORS

TOM KELSO, M.S., C.S.C.S., M.S.C.C.-E.

TK BOOKS
Terre Haute, Indiana

Cover designed by Phil Velikan

Printed in the United States of America
10 9 8 7 6 5 4 3 2 1

Packaged by
Wish Publishing
P.O. Box 10337
Terre Haute, IN 47801, USA
www.wishpublishing.com

"The time has come for someone to put his foot down
...and that foot is me."

Vernon Wormer
Dean of Students – Faber College
Circa 1978

TABLE OF CONTENTS

FOREWORD

There is much we know yet some we do not know about muscle contraction in resistance training. Past and on-going present research gives us a solid foundation with which to construct result-producing training programs, but we can always learn even more. From the days of solely barbells and dumbbells to more sophisticated equipment now found in training facilities, from outdated nutrition advice to a now better understanding of nutrient intake that compliments exercise prescriptions, and more time-efficient training methods that better fit into current day schedules of trainees, we've come a long way but have not reached the apex of perfection.

The intent of this book is to revisit the basics of what we currently know but then go a bit deeper into specific aspects of resistance training to better understand them, particularly things we've taken for granted or not taken the time to fully dissect.

By delving into some intricacies and aspects that have to date only been given a cursory glance, at the least it will hopefully confirm we are on the right track. At the most it is hoped it will stimulate thought and discussion that will lead to further research and refinement of existing resistance training exercise prescriptions.

By reading the entirety of this book these questions will be answered...

- How are muscles activated during a one repetition (rep) maximum (1-RM) compared to a 35-RM?

- What energy system(s) fuel the various number of reps that can be performed?

- Why do two people with the same body type and 1-RM differ in the number of reps performed to momentary muscle fatigue (MMF) with the same percentage of the 1-RM (i.e., 10 reps vs. 12 reps with 80%)?

- Is the quantity of motor units and muscle fibers (MUs/fibers) recruited and fatigued similar in any set to MMF regardless of the amount of resistance used and number of reps completed (i.e., light resistance x 20 reps vs. heavy resistance x eight reps)?

- Why is one able to perform additional reps following brief pauses during a set, usually holding the resistance in the locked-out/initial starting point of an exercise?

- What causes muscle failure in any set regardless if low reps or high reps are completed?

- Is there a value to performing single joint exercises as opposed to multi joint exercises due to MU/fiber differences between muscle groups?

- Why are some people freakishly strong while others are unfortunately very weak?

- Should all sets be performed to momentary muscle fatigue?

- What number of reps are most effective for increasing 1) strength, 2) power, 3) local muscle endurance, and 4) muscle size?

- Is there an optimal range of reps to perform based on one's genetic endowment?

- Which one is more important, the number of reps performed (i.e., 15) or the amount of time it takes to complete a set (i.e., :45)?

- Should multiple sets (i.e., two+) be performed for best results?

- Why does increasing muscle strength increase local muscle endurance?

- What are the optimal number of reps to perform when resistance training for fat loss?

Each of those questions will be answered specifically at the conclusion of all pertinent discussion.

Understanding the details of "what's going on in there?" in any resistance training scenario — whether using high or low reps, how muscles are contracting, the influence of muscle belly size, arm, and leg length, or the energy system is fueling the set — can offer better insight into personalizing a resistance training program whether the goal is becoming stronger, improving power, increasing muscle size, enhancing local muscle endurance, or even losing body fat.

BACKGROUND INFORMATION

To understand "what's going on in there?" during the performance of a resistance training set, it is prudent to grasp the underlying fundamentals of skeletal muscle composition, contraction, and other relevant factors. That would include discussion on:

1. Muscle fibers and motor units (MUs).

2. The nervous system.

3. Chemical interactions at the molecular level.

4. Energy systems fueling muscle.

5. Causes of fatigue.

6. Other genetic factors.

7. Training status and nutrition.

8. Skill acquisition and enhancement.

9. Motivation and mental toughness.

NOTE: So much research into the intricacies of muscle contraction have been limited in two ways: 1) the use of non-human muscle tissue to extrapolate findings from cats, frogs, goats (yes, goats), rabbits, rats, and other creatures) and 2) the use of small muscles in the human body (i.e., Adductor Pollicis [hand] and Soleus [smaller calf muscle], and many tests using isometric-only (static) contractions. The larger force-generating and locomotive muscles such as the Gluteals, Quadriceps, and Hamstrings along with shoulder girdle and upper limb muscles of humans — muscles more relevant to the study of performance (i.e., running, various sport skills, conventional resistance training) — *should* be studied more thoroughly. However, due to ethical, legal, and practical issues they are not.

ABBREVIATION KEY

The following is a list of important terms and abbreviations that will be used throughout this text:

1-, 10-, and 35-RM: A set of one rep, 10 reps, and 35 reps to momentary muscle fatigue (i.e., muscle "failure"), respectively.

2A: Intermediate MU/fiber type (between types 1 and 2X).

2X: Larger, faster, and less enduring MU/fiber type.

ADP: Adenosine diphosphate.

AP: Action potential.

ATP: Adenosine triphosphate.

Ca+: Calcium ions.

Cadence: The way a rep is performed.

CK: Creatine kinase.

CNS: Central nervous system.

Cr: Creatine.

GTO: Golgi Tendon Organ.

K: Potassium.

Mg: Magnesium.

MMF: Momentary muscle failure.

MN: Motor neuron.

MU: Motor unit.

MUs: Motor units.

MUs/fiber types: Motor units and its muscle fiber types.

MVC: Maximum voluntary contraction (voluntary = from the brain, not an outside mechanical source).

NA: Neurological ability.

NA/CNS potential: Same as NA, referencing one's central nervous system potential.

Na+: Sodium ions.

NJ: Neuromuscular junction.

P: Phosphate.

P = F x D/T: Formula for power output. Power equals force multiplied by distance divided by time.

PCr: Phosphocreatine, a.k.a., creatine phosphate.

Rep: Repetition.

Speed: The rate of movement, independent of direction.

SR: Sarcoplasmic reticulum.

Type 1: Smaller, slower, and more enduring MU/fiber type.

U. O. F.: Units of force generated by each of the three MU/fiber types.

Velocity: A vector quantity, the rate of change of speed in a certain direction.

MUSCLE CONTRACTION 101

Here is s a simple overview of "what's going in there?" from start to finish:

- A signal is sent to the muscles through the central nervous system (CNS). At each muscle fiber stimulated, or "recruited" a series of electro-chemical reactions occur at the neuromuscular junction (NJ).

- The actual contractile structures inside each muscle fiber – the sarcomeres that contain the interacting actin and myosin filaments - are activated.

- The actin and myosin create a "crossbridge" formation and collectively shorten the muscle belly.

- More chemical interaction occurs, the cross-bridging ceases, the muscle relaxes, and it returns to its original length.

That is the muscle contraction for dummies in a nutshell.

MUSCLE CONTRACTION 202

From the brain to the NJ a more detailed sequence of events that involve neuro-chemical-mechanical interaction and ultimately the actin and myosin cross-bridge force creation is as follows:

- It starts with that signal sent from the motor cortex of the brain to the spinal cord, to the motor neuron (MN), and finally to the motor unit (MU).

- The muscle fibers of the MU receive an action potential (AP) at the NJ, then it's transmitted via the T-tubules to the sarcoplasmic reticulum (SR).

- Acetylcholine is released into the sarcolemma. It depolarizes and sodium ions (Na+) enter the fiber and potassium (K) exits. This Sodium-Potassium "pump" is fueled by magnesium (Mg).

- Calcium ions (Ca+) are released from the SR terminal cisternae into the muscle sarcoplasm.

- Ca+ attach to the protein complex troponin. This unblocks tropomyosin and exposes the actin binding site.

- Adenosine diphosphate (ADP) adds a phosphate (P) and resynthesizes adenosine triphosphate (ATP). The thick myosin head binds to the thinner actin filament.

- The actin-myosin crossbridge forms and the thick myosin pulls on the thin actin filament. The result is the sarcomere shortens and the muscle contracts. The myosin head detaches when new ATP is hydrolyzed to ADP + P.

- The myosin head re-attaches and the process is repeated via the hydrolysis of ATP.

All that occurs from start to finish in all muscle fibers recruited, up to thousands of times, for the duration of a resistance training set lasting from a few seconds to many minutes. Imagine that also occurring in all active muscles during events ranging from short term (i.e., a discus throw) to long term (10 K run). It is fascinating stuff that is usually taken for granted.

To make this endeavor easier to understand regarding what is generally occurring in muscle during resistance training, some intricate details need to be discussed. However, to make it relatively easy to see the process when muscle tissue is activated to produce force and overcome resistance, examples of specific resistance training sets will be dissected to offer a clearer understanding of what's going on from the first to the last rep performed.

NOTE: Each forthcoming discussion section is presented with necessary intricate details to fully grasp its influence on contracting muscle during a resistance training set. Following each discussion is a — "So, Here's What's Important to Know" — section that summarizes key points.

1

MUSCLE FIBERS & MOTOR UNITS (MUs)

Muscle is comprised of many sub structures:

Entire muscle belly ➡ fascicles ➡ fibers ➡ myofibrils ➡ sarcomeres ➡ the myofilaments actin and myosin (see figure 1).

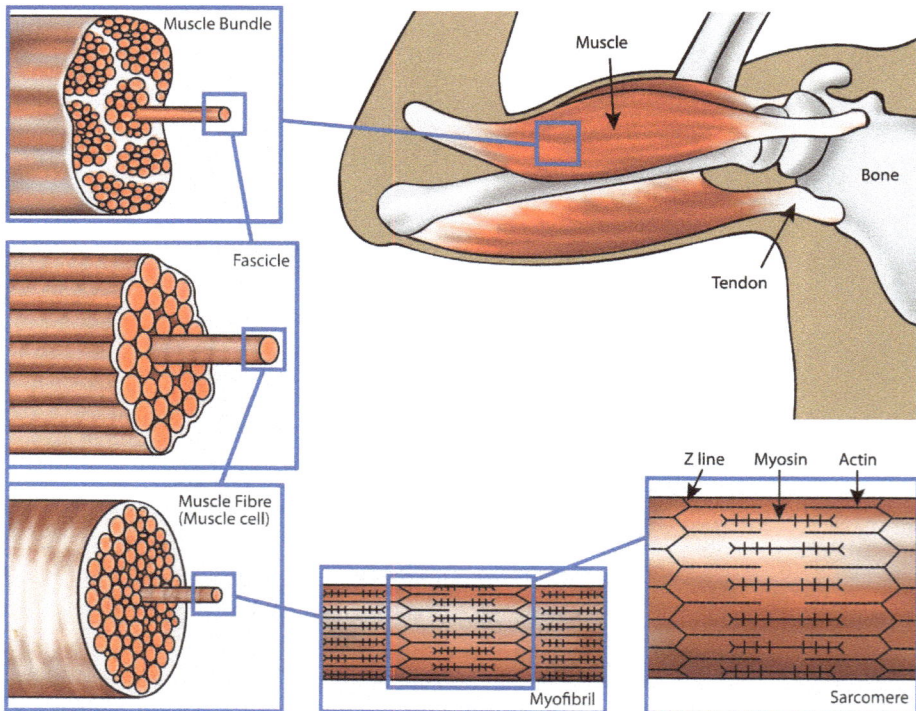

Figure 1: Entire Muscle and Substructures

Muscle fibers are the actual contracting structures within muscle. Fiber types fall on a continuum from smaller-weaker-slower contracting and more enduring on one end to larger-stronger-faster contracting and less enduring on the other. And it stands to reason that larger muscles (i.e., thighs) possess more fibers than small muscles (i.e., facial muscles) due to sheer volume.

It is common to discuss fiber types as either slow or fast when athletic performance and training program design are the topic. "He/she is explosive due to many fast fibers" or "Lifting light resistances will only develop your slow fibers" (which is actually not true). Generalizations, nonetheless.

Scientists in the first half of the 19th century initially classified muscle fibers as either red (oxidative, slower, more capillaries) or white (less oxidative, faster, less capillaries). It wasn't until the mid-20th century when more advanced methods allowed for more distinctive classification into three types: 1) more oxidative, more enduring, and relatively smaller in size 2) less oxidative, less enduring, and relatively larger in size, and 3) an intermediate type which had some characteristics of each of those.

Interestingly, it was not until the late 1980s that a fourth type of muscle fiber was discovered — one that functioned between the intermediate and less oxidative type — and was labeled type IIB (see four categories below). Even more recently, researchers further made a distinction between the collection of the faster-to-fatigue/less oxidative fibers and added a fifth type as noted below.

Three methods are now used to specifically classify fiber types based on their: 1) myosin ATPase (enzyme) activity, 2) myosin heavy chain (MHC) isoform, and 3) total metabolic capacity. (1)

Regarding fiber-type classification systems, the categories that have been used over the years are as follows, from the smaller/weaker/slower/more enduring on the left to the larger/stronger/faster/less enduring on the right:

Three categories:

- SO (slow oxidative) – FOG (fast oxidative glycolic) – FG (fast glycolytic)
- MHC I (myosin heavy chain 1) - MHC IIA - MHC IIX
- S (slow) – FFR (fast fatigue resistant) – FF (fast fatigable)

Four categories:

- SO (slow oxidative) – FI (fast intermediate) – FR (fast fatigue resistant) – FF (fast fatigable)
- I - IIA – IIB – IIC (2)

Five categories:

• 1 – 1/2A – 2A – 2A/B – 2B (3)

Because there are functional differences between muscle fibers (and corresponding motor units), to simplify all further discussion they will be classified into three types: type **1**, type **2A**, and type **2X**. The type 1 will be the smaller, weaker, but more enduring. Type 2X will be the opposite: larger, stronger, but less enduring. Type 2A will be that intermediate fiber in the middle that possesses characteristics of the other two. In that way a reasonable distinction of each will be set and better help explain the resistance training examples used throughout this book.

Regarding the three types of muscle fibers and their functions, type 2A intermediate and fast 2X fibers contract a bit faster than slow type 1 fibers – and consequently have that less endurance. Also, type 2A intermediate and 2X fast are larger and stronger than slow type 1 and are called upon when more strength/force generation is needed.

Understand, though, even though slow, intermediate, and fast refer to their contraction speed, more significantly it depicts their endurance capacity. That is, slow type 1 fibers have more endurance (i.e., lower force, lengthy activities such as walking) and fast type 2X fibers have less endurance (i.e., higher force, short-duration activities such as heavy lifting). Type 2A intermediate fibers are a bit closer in function to type 2X but can adapt to function to an extent like Type 1 (or type 2X) depending on the training stimulus applied to them. For example, if the type 2A fibers are exposed to longer, more enduring exercise they improve their capacity for that. And if trained with short-term high force stimuli they will adapt toward improving that ability.

NOTE: Local muscle endurance should not be confused with the cardiovascular endurance, respiratory endurance, or general muscle endurance, all of which pertain to the entire body's ability to perform over an extended period. Local muscle endurance is the ability of one specific muscle group or a small group of muscles performing a specific exercise for an extended period (i.e., for more reps). In example, performing a pull/chin up involves the elbow flexors, shoulder extensors and adductors, and scapula adductors. Improving local muscle endurance in those muscle groups would allow for more pull/chin up reps to be performed.

In addition, the size differential between type 1 and both type 2 fibers can be a factor, especially when the goal is increasing muscle size (hypertrophy). Because they are relatively larger, a person possessing more type 2X and 2A fibers in a specific muscle belly has the better potential to increase the size of that muscle when compared to a person lacking that, especially when there is a large discrepancy between the quantity of smaller type 1 and larger type 2 fibers.

Regarding muscle volume one's body type must also be considered. Imagine a continuum with one end being endomorphic (short & round) and on the other end ectomorphic (tall and thin). Somewhere between is the mesomorphic body type (muscular and lean). Everyone is somewhere on that continuum, either one type or a combination of types.

The key is the amount of muscle mass one possesses. All other factors being equal, the greater the muscle mass, the greater the quantity of fibers. Short and round body types – even though they may have above average limb and torso girth measurements - may contain more body fat and less muscle. Tall and thin will possess longer muscle bellies but most likely less overall muscle mass. The mesomorphic stocky muscular type obviously has more relative muscle mass, thus more fibers, hence more strength potential (see figure 2).

NOTE: When the phrase "All other factors being equal" is mentioned from here on out, it means the discussed factor by itself would either positively or negatively affect an outcome or process. That is, factors A, B, and C may each be an advantage or disadvantage, but the influence of the specific factor B is the only variable to consider in that instance.

Another significant factor is the quantity of muscle fiber types relative to each other. One may possess an average quantity of all three types, but another may possess an above average or below average quantity of one specific type which affects the proportion of the other two. An example would be possessing a below average quantity of type 1, average quantity of type 2A, and an above average quantity of type 2X fibers in the hamstrings.

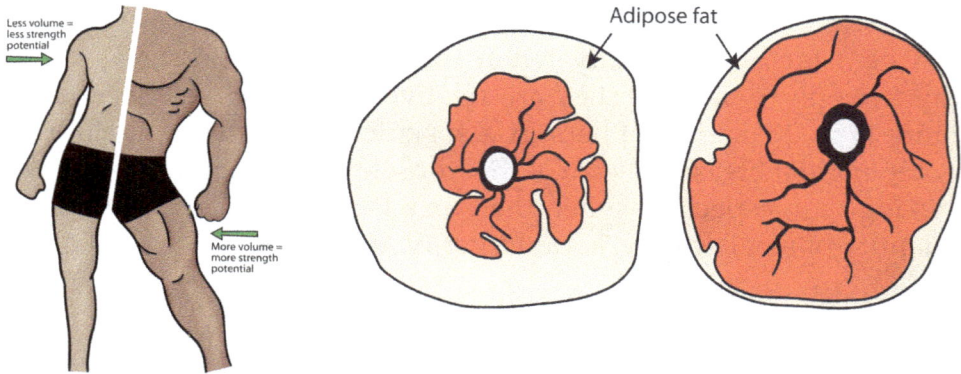

Figure 2: Muscle Volume Difference – More Mass = More Strength Potential

Various possibilities exist regarding the quantity and proportion of type 1, type 2A, and type 2X fibers relative to each. That fact explains why some people have unusual ability in certain activities. A small muscled person will have fewer total fibers but may possess an above average quantity of type 2X and thus the ability to exert exceptional strength. Likewise, a large-muscled person will naturally have more total fibers combined but may possess an above average quantity of type 1 fibers (thus relatively fewer type 2 fibers), and therefore only able to exert average strength.

Fiber type distribution can also vary between different muscle groups and impact resistance training exercise performance. Between two people, in example, both may possess an average quantity of all fiber types in their deltoids, but one may possess a below average quantity of 2X and above average quantity of type 1 in the triceps. This person would be (all other factors being equal) at a disadvantage strength-wise when comparing ability in an overhead press exercise.

Another example would be a wide grip pulldown performance and the involved biceps and latissimus dorsi muscles. One's biceps may possess an average quantity of type 1, above average type 2A, and below average type 2X, but their middle and inferior regions of the latissimus dorsi may possess a below average quantity of type 1, average type 2A, and above average type 2X. How would that affect prescribing appropriate exercise prescriptions for the pulldown to maximally train those muscles?

With so many possible combinations and differences between all people – varied muscle volume, the proportion of each fiber type, and differences between individual muscle groups - it can be confounding when comparing results and designing one-size-fits-all training plans. Just remember that all other factors being equal, a smaller person who possesses an above average quantity of smaller type 1 should be able to out-perform a larger person with an above average quantity of larger type 2X when engaging in a long duration/low force event such as a 10K run. Conversely, the larger and above average type 2X person should have an advantage in a weightlifting or bodybuilding contest as compared to the smaller and above average type 1 person.

Ultimately, it all comes down to the total quantity of a specific fiber type that more significantly effects the performance between two people, all other factors being equal. Keep that in mind as we move forward.

Motor units: A MU is a group of the same muscle fiber type connected to a motor neuron (MN) in the CNS. It is the MU and its corresponding individual fibers that receive a signal from the CNS to ultimately contract muscle to generate force. Generally, the more MUs recruited means more force can be exerted.

NOTE: The MNs ➡ MUs ➡ individual muscle fibers order is the "structural' sequence in the CNS signaling order. Therefore, when the terms slow or fast, type 1, type 2A, or type 2X, or MU(s)/ fibers are used to distinguish MU/fiber characteristics in any forthcoming discussion, the MU, MN, and fiber type are all one in the same (i.e., type 2A MNs = type 2A MUs = type 2A fibers).

Just as larger muscles contain more individual fibers as compared to smaller muscles, it follows that larger muscles contain more MUs than smaller muscles. In example, the medial gastrocnemius (calf muscle) may have 579 MUs that control a total of 1,120,000 individual muscle fibers @ 1,934 fibers per MU. The First Dorsal Interosseous (hand muscle) may have 119 MUs that control a total of 40,500 individual muscle fibers @ 340 fibers per MU. (4)

Regarding how MUs are distributed in muscle tissue:

- Muscle fibers attached to the same MU unit are usually arranged throughout the entire muscle belly in a mosaic-type pattern.

- In addition, only few muscle fibers from the same MU lie immediately adjacent to each other.

- On that, the distribution of fibers in single MUs is normally random.

- Regardless of how they populate muscle tissue, their arrangement must comply with the whole muscle belly to produce meaningful force patterns.

A Brief Discussion on Muscle Spindles and Golgi Tendon Organs (GTO) Within the Neuromuscular Dystem. (5)

Even though muscle spindles and GTOs play a sub-role in muscle contraction during conventional resistance training exercises, their importance is more predominant when fast speeds of contraction come into play. This would include activities such as sprinting and jumping, and as an injury defense mechanism protecting skeletal joints from being compromised. Additionally, they play a role in central (CNS) fatigue that will be touched on later. Therefore, it is prudent to at least know their existence and functions, but the focus of this book is on the more superficial contractile muscle tissue in the fascicles: the fibers connected to MUs and their contracting myofilaments (refer to figure 1).

Muscle Spindles: The muscle fibers that contract and allow the skeletal muscles to move the bones are termed extrafusal. Other sensory-type fibers contained within skeletal muscle – muscle spindles - are termed intrafusal. Intrafusal muscle spindles signal 1) the current length and 2) change of length of skeletal muscle. Muscle spindles are a collection of six to eight specialized fibers, and further classified into three types:

1. **Nuclear Chain** – their nuclei are aligned in single row & convey information on the static length of muscle.

2. **Static Nuclear Bag** – their nuclei are bundled in the middle of the fiber and too convey the static length of muscle.

3. **Dynamic Nuclear Bag** – their nuclei are bundled like the static nuclear bag fibers but convey information on the rate of change (velocity) of the length of muscle.

Fine, precise movement muscles such as the finger muscles have many spindles. Larger muscles that are responsible for body posture/gross movements have fewer spindles.

Golgi Tendon Organs: Golgi Tendon Organs (GTO) are another type of sensory fiber. They are located between skeletal muscle and corresponding tendons that attach to bones.

GTOs are arranged in a series pattern with muscle fibers and convey signals about the load or force experienced by the muscle. They are made of collagen fibers and innervated by *intrafusal* receptor type Ib fibers (different than the main contracting *extrafusal* types 1, 2A, and 2X fibers). Essentially, a certain amount of force stretches the GTO, the collagen fibers pinch the membranes of Ib fiber sensory endings, the Ib fibers depolarize and elicit action potentials, and ultimately signal the load/force amount.

— So, Here's What's Important to Know —

1. Larger muscles contain more muscle fibers and consequently more motor units (MUs) as compared to smaller muscles.

2. On the smaller type 1 to larger type 2X MU/fiber continuum, type 1 are weaker, have more endurance, and contract slower relative to the stronger, less enduring, and faster contracting type 2A and 2X MUs/fibers.

3. MUs/fibers are distributed randomly in a mosaic-type pattern throughout muscle bellies and can vary in proportion from one muscle group to another.

4. In general, a person with a greater quantity of MUs/fibers of a specific type may have a distinct performance advantage over a person with a lesser quantity of the same type, all other factors being equal (more on this later).

5. Other sensory fibers – muscle spindles and Golgi Tendon Organs – are contained within muscle tissue and provide feedback in the CNS. However, their functions are beyond the scope of this book.

2

THE NERVOUS SYSTEM

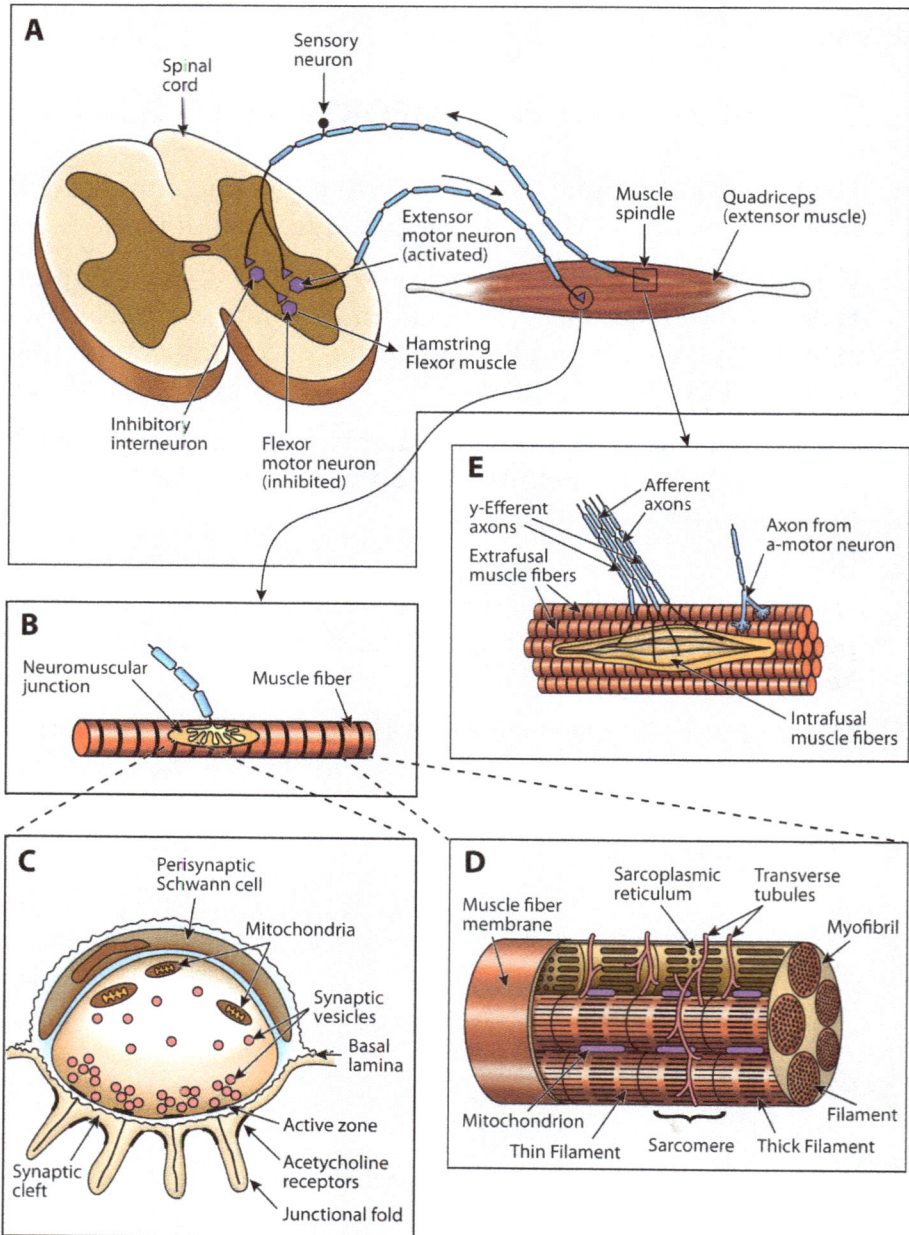

Figure 3: Overview of Neural Command of Muscle Fibers

The CNS governs MU control depending on the desired muscle force output. Essentially there are two means by which this occurs:

1. An orderly recruitment from low threshold type 1 to high threshold type 2X MUs/fibers via the Henneman's Size Principle.

2. Rate coding of signals sent through the CNS to the recruited MUs/fibers.

In general, figure 4 depicts the MU/fiber type recruitment scheme based on the level of force required to perform a task:

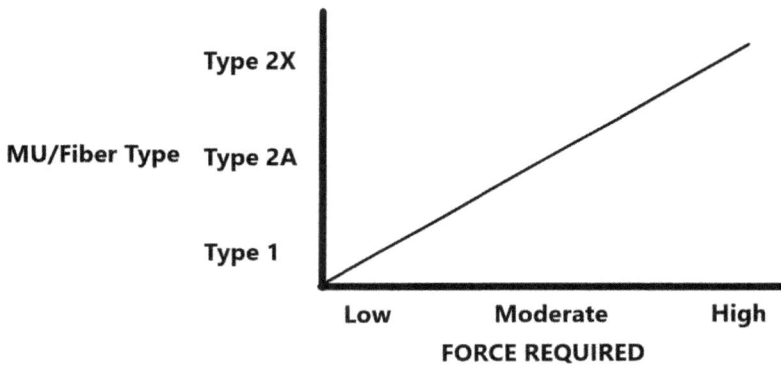

Figure 4: Basic Muscle Force and MU/Fiber Recruitment Scheme

Henneman's Size Principle

Regardless of the amount of force needed, the Henneman's Size Principle of MU recruitment is king (Henneman's Principle from this point forward). The principle states that MUs are always recruited from the smallest to the largest, or lower threshold to higher threshold. That is, if it is an easy low force task, the smaller and slower type 1 MUs are activated to do the job. As the force demand increases, the harder-to-turn on type 2A MUs are called upon. Then, if needed, highest threshold type 2X MUs are activated. In most resistance training events high force output/effort is required at some point. Therefore, the activation of all MU/fiber types usually occurs with each type contributing proportionally depending on the amount force needed to complete the task.

Think of it in this manner: pushing or pulling a small child's wagon loaded with light-weight plastic toys can be accomplished with minimal force generated by a single person. To push or pull a large cargo wagon loaded with scrap iron requires maximal force and the need for multiple people to accomplish the task. Bottom line: low force = less MUs required and high force = more MUs required.

Most small muscles recruit all MUs via Henneman's Principle at approximately 50% maximum voluntary contraction (MVC). Think small muscles (fingers and facial muscles) and think finer, precise movements.

Most large muscles increase force via Henneman's Principle up to 85% MVC. Think large muscles (gluteals, latissimus dorsi) and think larger, gross movements (i.e., running, pull ups).

The low force requirements people experience throughout the day (i.e., walking, reaching for something, rising from a sitting position) can be completed with the lower-threshold type 1 MUs/fibers. In instances where a greater demand is present and a higher force is required (i.e., lifting a heavy container, resistance training), one must dig into the higher threshold type 2A and 2X (if needed) MUs/fibers to successfully complete the task.

RATE CODING

Muscle contraction can also be regulated through the process called rate coding. The CNS network can upgrade or downgrade muscle force by varying the rate coding of already activated, or "recruited" MUs/fibers. Rate coding is the rate at which action potentials (AP) discharge to contract muscles. In more detail, a single AP from a motor neuron will produce a single contraction – a "twitch" - in the muscle fibers of its motor unit. Each muscle fiber twitch involves three phases: (6)

PHASE 1: LATENT PERIOD.

The time when the AP is spreading along the sarcolemma and calcium ions (Ca^+) are released from the SR. At this point excitation and contraction are being coupled but no contraction has occurred yet.

PHASE 2: CONTRACTION.

The actual contraction of muscle occurs when Ca^+ in the sarcoplasm have attached to troponin causing tropomyosin to move from the actin binding sites, thus allowing a cross-bridge to form. Here the sarcomeres actively shorten to create peak tension, the visible muscle shortening that occurs when lifting a resistance.

PHASE 3: RELAXATION.

Following the contraction process the tension decreases to a point of complete stoppage. Ca^+ are pumped out of the sarcoplasm and back into the SR and cross-bridging ends. The muscle fibers now return to their resting state.

SUMMATION OF FORCE

Using a low force contraction example, here is how force increases via Henneman's Principle and rate coding working together. It is essentially a progressive process that adds more force to each prior force produced:

1. An AP occurs in MU 1 to produce a slight twitch at a steady rate of 5 Hertz (Hz), then it relaxes (more on Hz forthcoming).

2. When MU 1 fires again and reaches 10 Hz, a 2nd AP occurs in MU 2 at the same 5 Hz twitch force.

3. MUs 1 and 2 increase their firing frequencies, until MU 1 reaches about 15 Hz and MU 2 about 10 Hz.

4. At this point, MU 3 is activated, and it continues in this manner by recruiting new MUs serially by adding 5 Hz to the firing frequency of previously recruited MUs. (7)

5. The key to this progressive force is the constant supply of Ca+ that needs to be present for actin-myosin cross-bridging. Continual "dumping" of Ca+ into the sarcoplasm from more frequent APs allows for faster twitches (rate coding) of each fiber.

6. With increasing APs/firing rates, a summation of force increases up to a point where it flatlines. At this point the muscle is experiencing maximum CNS potential in both recruitment and rate coding, a display called fused tetanus. (see figure 5).

Fused tetanus is the maximum ability to recruit muscle force within one's neurological ability/central nervous system (NA/CNS potential) that will be discussed in the Other Genetic Factors section.

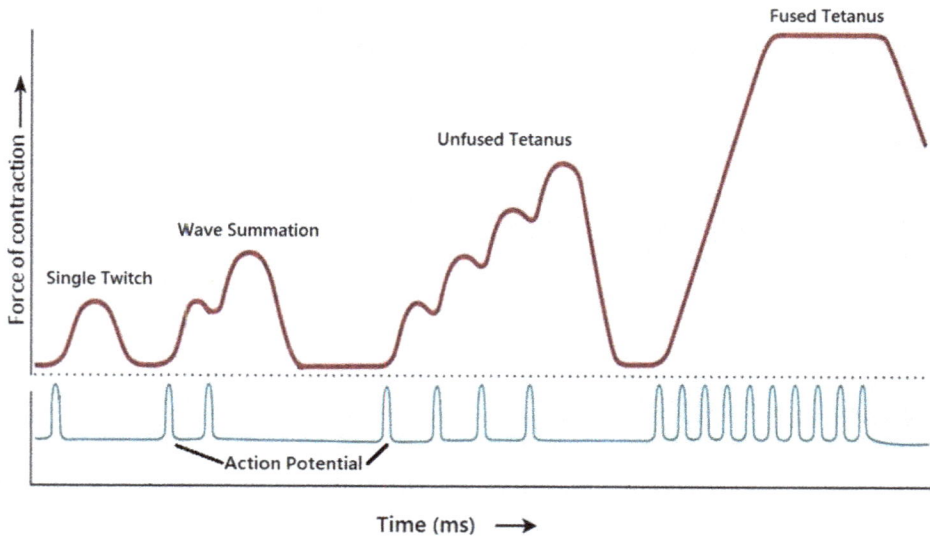

Figure 5: Fused Tetanus (8)

Summary of the process from low force to high force demands (if more force is needed, move to the next step):

1. Recruit the smaller, lower-enduring, lower threshold type 1 MUs/fibers.

2. Recruit more type 1.

3. Increase the rate coding of type 1.

4. Recruit the intermediate type 2A MUs/fibers.

5. Recruit more type 2A.

6. Increase the rate coding of type 2A.

7. Recruit the larger, less-enduring, higher threshold type 2X MUs/fibers.

8. Recruit more type 2X.

9. Increase the rate coding of type 2X.

10. Full tetanus is now achieved within one's NA/CNS potential.

CONTRACTION SPEED

Regarding muscle contraction speed, it is measured in Hertz (Hz) and milliseconds (ms). Hertz is a derived unit of frequency. One Hz is equal to one cycle-vibration-pulse per second (s). One second is equal to 1,000 ms. The greater the Hz, the faster the contraction (lesser ms).

As the firing rate increases, the time interval between APs decreases. In example, a single MU firing at 6 Hz may have an interval between APs of 166 ms. When the firing increases to 12 Hz, the interval between APs may decrease to 85 ms. (7)

Here are a few examples of muscles and their contraction speed potential. Note the average MU/fiber type quantity and contraction speed in Hz:

Biceps Brachii - high quantity of type 2 MUs @ 31.1 Hz

Adductor Pollicis (hand) - high quantity of type 2 MUs @ 29.9 Hz

Soleus (calf) - high quantity of type 1 MUs @ 10.7 Hz

Tibialis Anterior (shin) – high quantity of type 2 MUs @ 32.1 Hz

Type 1 MUs/fibers – the slowest of all - contract in the range of 90 to 140 ms, or .09 to .14 seconds (s). That is still fast when it comes to human movement. Type 2A contract faster (50 to 100 ms/.05 to .1 s) and type 2X even a bit faster (40 to 90 ms/.04 to .09 s). (7). Not much difference between 2A and 2X MUs/fibers, but more of a difference between type 2 and type 1.

What accounts for the earlier recruitment of type 1/slow and not the type 2/fast MUs/fibers? Know that a form of electrical current – specifically the flow of ions – runs through the central nervous system to trigger muscle contraction. And that flow of ions is all about Ohm's Law.

Ohm's Law: the current (ion) flow in AMPS = voltage (across a conductor) ÷ resistance (in OHMS). (9)

Type 1/slow MNs have a smaller membrane surface and fewer ion channels, therefore a higher input resistance. Type 2 MNs have a greater membrane surface and more ion channels, therefore a lower input resistance. So, regarding OHM's Law, a lower amount of current input at the neuromuscular junction (NJ) is enough for the type 1/slow MUs/ fibers to reach firing threshold while the type 2/fast MUs/fibers will remain below the threshold. With more electrical current – that is, the higher the MN stimulation – the greater the type 2/fast MU fiber activation.

Even though there is a slight difference between each MU/fiber type, all contract relatively fast in under 14/100ths of a second. The point to make here is even type 1/slow MUs/fibers are involved in moving the body fast in situations unabated by resistance.

Take a vertical jump, a quick hop, throwing a punch, or kicking a football. All are executed initially with the assistance of the categorical "easier-to-turn-on" type 1 slow MUs/fibers along with a certain quantity of type 2A and 2X in those short-term events (both type 2 MUs/fibers being more difficult to turn on). Remember the Henneman's Principle order of recruitment that must be followed: 1 ➡ 2A ➡ 2X. Because the aforementioned events involve moving the limbs against minimal resistance (i.e., weight of shoes, a football, or boxing gloves) the majority of work is initially completed by the type 1 MUs/fibers, and then a quantity of type 2A ➡ 2X near the end of the event based on the need of additional force, if any (relative to the force-velocity curve to be addressed later). Their activation may only be minimal due to the greater time it takes to turn them on (READ: Ohm's Law).

To sum that up, in many non-resisted, quick, and brief actions, the slow type 1 MUs/fibers are involved, and not exclusively the fast type 2. In resistance training, however, many MUs/fibers from type 1 through type 2X are recruited due to the fact significant resistance is used, even in conventional high rep/low resistance sets (i.e., 55% to 70% of an equivalent 1-RM, which is still 55% to 70% greater than zero resistance). As reps are completed in succession – and a progressive recruitment of MUs/fibers via the Henneman's Principle occurs due to the fatigue of the prior recruited MUs/fibers and need to continue force output - a large number will have been recruited and overloaded (fatigued) at the point of momentary muscle fatigue, especially in relatively higher rep sets.

OTHER FACTORS

Force-Velocity Relationship. The force output and velocity (rate of change relative to position and time) of muscle contraction varies: As muscle velocity increases the force output declines (see figure 6).

On the left side of the figure, force (blue line) is maximum because velocity is zero. There is also no power (red line) displayed because power = force x velocity (and no velocity exists). An example of this would be an all-out isometric contraction against an immovable object.

On the right side the reverse is true: At maximum velocity, no force is generated because actin-myosin cross-bridging cannot occur. This also results in zero power. An example of this would be the end of the action of throwing a ¼ pound object. The greatest amount of relative force was already created during the initial throwing movements, as noted by the bisecting green dotted line. Maximum power is created at approximately the one-third point of the maximum shortening velocity of the involved muscles.

Applying this to resistance training performance is simple: A heavy resistance creates the need for maximum force creation (maximum MU/fiber recruitment, type 1➡ 2A ➡ 2X). However, a heavy resistance cannot be moved relatively fast (gravitational pull, thank you Sir Isaac Newton). Lighten the resistance significantly and the velocity increases, but less force is created due to the lower the demand and faster movement.

Understand it is all relative to one's maximum strength. All other factors being equal, the stronger one is the faster they can move a lighter resistance. In example, person with a 1-RM of 300 pounds would be able to move 30% of that resistance – 90 pounds – much faster than a person with a 1-RM of only 200 pounds. For the 200/1-RM person, 90 pounds would represent 45% of the 1-RM, a relatively heavier resistance, and the inability to move it at the same velocity. It is simple physics.

At this point a few questions come to mind regarding the optimal resistance training loads and the efforts required to move (lift) them:

1. Is it better to use very heavy resistances and attempt to move them as fast as possible even though they will not move fast?

2. What about lighter loads and movement intents? Slow and controlled (when they could be moved relatively fast) or as fast as possible and for as many reps possible?

More on that forthcoming.

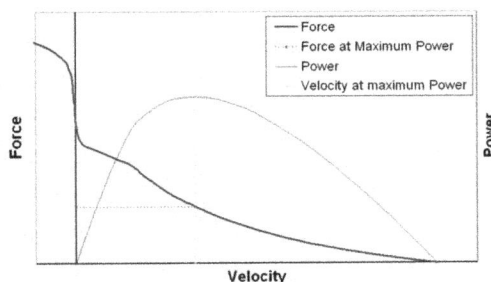

Figure 6: Force-Velocity (10)

MU/fiber Reserve. A 1-RM effort requires all available MUs/fibers to complete it. Once completed, a second rep is not possible due to the fatigue of some, but not all, of the higher-threshold MUs/fibers. Many are unfatigued, but the number available is below the maximum number required, hence the event must end.

In submaximal efforts such as long-duration, extended sets of 12, 20, or 30+ reps, MUs/fibers work on a "substitution/rotation" basis. Fewer MUs/fibers are required initially to move a submaximal resistance through each rep of the exercise's range of motion. Therefore, some are recruited, and others are not. This offers a MU/fiber reserve that is available to complete multiple reps as fatigue gradually takes its toll during the event (11). This is essentially the local muscle endurance ability/quality previously mentioned.

Units of force. This must be clearly understood to grasp the force output of the three MU/fibers types when moving any amount of resistance during a set. Recall type 1 MUs/fibers are smaller and weaker as compared to the intermediate type 2A (larger and stronger than type 1) and type 2X (even larger and stronger than type 2A). Therefore, it's not solely the number of total MUs/fibers recruited, but the amount of force each type generates. In example, 100 type 2X MUs/fibers generate a greater amount of force as compared to 100 type 1 MUs/fibers and this significantly affects the recruitment and fatigue process from the first to the last rep.

In forthcoming examples and descriptions, a unit of force (U. O. F.) will be assigned to each MU/fiber type to simplify discussion, as follows:

Type 1 = 1 U. O. F.

Type 2A = 2 U. O. F.

Type 2X = 3 U. O. F.

Therefore, 500 type 1 MUs/fibers would have a total of 500 U. O. F., 500 2A would have 1,000 U. O. F., and 500 2X would have 1,500 U. O. F.

A resistance capable of being moved for 20 reps to muscle fatigue may only require 930 U. O. F. each rep even though a combined total of 1,350 "recruitable" U. O. F. is available (all MU/fiber types combined). The unrecruited are a part of the reserve pool. As reps are subsequently performed and the set becomes more difficult, other MUs/fibers must be called upon (the reserve) to assist and/or replace the previously recruited MUs/fibers (some fatigued/some not). Understand it always requires a certain quantity of U. O. F. coming from a combination of all

MU/fiber types to move the 20-RM resistance, so more must be added as fatigue accrues over the completion of reps in the set. At the point of MMF at the conclusion of the 20th rep, one is unable to recruit enough U. O. F. to add to the 930 total pool required to perform a now impossible 21st rep.

Understanding the U. O. F. contribution of each MU/fiber type is critical when dissecting the recruitment and fatigue process in all resistance training sets regardless of the number of reps performed. The detailed explanation of the forthcoming 1-RM, 10-RM, and 35-RM diagrams will clearly depict the connection between MU/fiber types, their U. O. F., and the reserve U. O. F. from the start (unfatigued) to completion (MMF) of each RM set.

70% Rule. A complete recruitment of every single MU/fiber in the network is a rarity, and only occurs in odd situations (see NOTES box below). Research has determined that muscles artificially stimulated could produce more force output when compared to a person's MVC via their conscious effort to recruit a maximum quantity. The optimum stimulation rate needed to create maximum contraction ranges from 50 to 100 Hz but maximum frequencies measured in MVC of most muscles fall short of that range (12).

A study using dynamic magnetic resonance imaging determined, on average, approximately 70% of all available MUs/fibers can be recruited in any conscious MVC (13). So, in any MVC event, one can recruit on average only 70% of their 100% total quantity of all MUs/fibers in the involved muscles. It seems odd, but imagine exerting maximum, gut-wrenching effort when trying to lift the back end of a car or performing a 1-RM leg press. You'd only be using 70% of all the MUs/fibers you possessed leaving 30% "unrecruited" in that 100% effort.

There can be, however, exceptions as some may possess an above average (i.e., 73%) or below average (i.e., 66%) ability. Even though slight above or slight below the 70% average, small differences can significantly affect individual abilities and outcomes regarding the amount of resistances used in resistance training sets and the number of reps possible with various percentages of a 1-RM (more on this in the NA/CNS potential discussion in the Other Genetic Factors section).

NOTE: A complete voluntary recruitment of every single MU/ muscle fiber contained in the involved muscles does not occur due to the built-in defense mechanism that protects against joint/ muscle injury. It also allows for a reserve supply for extended work within the confines of both central and peripheral fatigue factors. A simultaneous recruitment of all MUs/fibers occurs only when 1) a person is electrocuted, 2) artificial stimulation is provided in vitro, or 3) a person is facing a rare life or death situation and CNS inhibition is bypassed. Proof that muscle and joint damage will result can be seen in cases where accidental electrocution occurs. (2, 14)

Modes of Contraction and MVC. Regarding the MVC of different contractions modes, MU/fiber recruitment in eccentric (negative/ lowering) contractions is greater than in concentric (positive/raising) contractions. That is why more resistance can be lowered under control against gravity than lifted upward against gravity. During isometric (static) contractions, pure constant force is impossible due to the oscillation of the actin-myosin cross-bridging. High static force is capable of being generated, but it occurs at a lower frequency of MU/fiber recruitment.

Regardless of the contraction mode, all three can be used productively in a well-designed resistance training program.

Rep Performance: Eccentric & Concentric Phases, Velocity & Cadence, and ATP Usage. Regarding the performance of each rep in a set - more specifically the concentric and eccentric phases – it is the repeated performance of each rep that ultimately leads to the desired goal of the set. Therefore, knowledge of "what's going on in there" during a complete rep cycle from start to finish is critical so the entire collection of accumulated reps leads to the intended results.

In the **concentric phase** (muscle shortening/resistance raising) only the active elements are at work. That would be the interaction of actin and myosin in the cross-bridging process. When cross-bridging occurs, the sarcomere shortens due to a greater overlap. However, muscle is weaker, and more ATP must be used as compared to the eccentric phase. Because they need to "work harder" and rely on more ATP concentrically, the potential for greater fatigue occurs due to greater metabolite accumulation. In addition, as fatigue increases, the velocity of contraction decreases. This progressive fatigue increases the mechanical loading on the MUs/fibers and the result is greater force output relative to the force-velocity relationship (15).

In the **eccentric phase** (muscle lengthening/resistance lowering) both the active and passive elements are at work. Along with the active actin and myosin elements, the addition of the passive elements Titin, the fiber cytoskeleton, and surrounding endomysium components also assist. They possess elastic qualities that resist overall muscle stretch. As a result, muscle is stronger, more resistance can be used, and less ATP is required as compared to the concentric phase. The active actin and myosin elements are now detaching to allow for the muscle to lengthen, hence the less ATP required (16).

The **Velocity and Cadence** of a rep is also critical for optimal development. A goal in rep performance is to create tension in the muscle fibers to produce high force output. Recall that moving a resistance too fast decreases overall MU/fiber recruitment, lowers tension, and lessens force output as the emphasis shifts to the right on the force/velocity curve. Therefore, moving resistance slower and under control (i.e., no jerking, yanking, excessive momentum-creating actions) is desirable. But remember it is called resistance training for a reason. Significant resistance must be used to glean any benefit, thus 1) relatively heavy resistances must be used (i.e., 55% to 100% of a 1-RM) which cannot in themselves be moved relatively fast to begin with and 2) when an appropriate resistance is used that has the potential to be moved faster (i.e., 55%), it must consciously be moved under control, creating maximum tension relative to its amount.

So, it all comes down to what is a meaningful velocity and cadence during both the concentric and eccentric phases of a rep. The prudent advice is if in doubt slow it down. Think controlled effort on the concentric phase, use control on the eccentric phase (i.e., do not drop the resistance), and when fatigue begins to naturally slow overall velocity, think explode concentrically and keep resisting in the eccentric phase. That will maximize MU/fiber recruitment. In the latter more-fatiguing stages of a set worked to MMF, it is actually the safest part of the set due to the naturally slower velocity and inability to create excess momentum, something that could compromise both muscle and connective tissue integrity.

— So, Here's What's Important to Know —-

1. MUs and their muscle fibers are recruited by the central nervous system via 1) the Henneman's Principle (smaller to larger type, depending on the amount of force needed) and 2) Rate Coding (their firing rate).

2. In general, low force requires less MU/fiber recruitment and high force requires more MU/fiber activation.

3. Type 1 MUs/fibers have both a longer contraction time and twitch duration while type 2 MUs/fibers have both a shorter contraction time and twitch duration.

4. Even though type 1 MUs/fibers contract slower by only a few milliseconds as compared to both type 2 MUs/fibers, they are responsible for the many quick body weight-only movements in daily life, such as an explosive hop, an urgent rise from a seated position, or a quick upward reach with the hand.

5. MUs/fibers in smaller muscles usually reach complete recruitment around 50% of maximum voluntary contraction (MVC) and then rely on a faster rate coding to increase force to a certain level. Larger muscles reach complete recruitment around 85% MVC and then use faster rate coding to reach full CNS potential.

6. Rate coding helps regulate muscle force output as it increases the firing rate of all recruitable MUs/fibers in a coordinated manner to create a summation of force display within one's respective NA/CNS potential.

7. That maximum potential is deemed neurological ability (NA) and amounts to an average of 70% of the total number of MUs/fibers that can be activated at any one instance. The ability to recruit and fire the greatest number of MUs/fibers is called maximum fused tetanus.

8. MUs/fiber types have different levels of force generation potential to add to the force requirement of the event. For the sake of all forthcoming discussion, type 1 (smallest/weakest) have been assigned a "unit of force" (U. O. F.) value of 1, type 2A (intermediate size and strength) a value of 2, and type 2X (largest/strongest) a value of 3.

9. Regarding the force-velocity curve and the law of gravitational pull, the heavier the resistance, the slower it will move relative to one's maximum strength. Conversely, the velocity of movement increases as the amount of resistance decreases.

10. More force is generated via muscle fiber cross-bridging with heavier resistances and/or with lighter resistances as velocity slows due to the onset of fatigue. Therefore, for optimal rep performance and force generation, use a controlled movement cadence and velocity.

11. Eccentric/lowering contractions recruit more MUs/fibers, are stronger, and use less ATP as compared to concentric/raising and isometric/static contractions.

3

CHEMICAL REACTIONS AT THE MOLECULAR LEVEL

The structural components of muscle contraction are the brain, axon, sensory organs, MUs, and all attached muscle fibers including their sarcomeres. They require certain chemicals to carry out the entire contraction process. Akin to an automobile needing electricity from a battery, gasoline, oil, brake fluid, anti-freeze, etc. to properly and safely move it from point A to B, these chemical compounds must be present at various points from the start/contraction to the finish/relaxation.

The minerals sodium (Na) and potassium (K) are essential for proper nerve function. Both Na and K help the nerve cells send electrical signals to create an action potential at the NJ to initiate muscle contraction.

The minerals calcium (Ca) and magnesium (Mg) are needed for the actual mechanism of both muscle fiber contraction and relaxation. They interact with the protein filaments actin and myosin which ultimately perform those actions. The actin and myosin rely on Ca to engage and cross-bridge, and on Mg to relax after a contraction occurs.

The molecule adenosine triphosphate (ATP) is the ultimate necessity for muscle contraction. ATP must be present at various sites during the process and if not available, no contraction occurs.

ATP is the main energy source of all cells in the body. More discussion on this later but know ATP in the body comes from dietary intake, which ultimately comes from sunlight via photosynthesis in plants: Eat vegetables, fruit, and nuts = get ATP. Eat proteins and fats from living creatures that also consumed those plants = get ATP. Eat protein and fats from living creatures that consumed other living creatures that consumed those plants = get ATP. So, thank sunlight for the ability to move the body from one point to another.

Three locations require ATP to fully complete the entire contraction process:

1. At the actin-myosin binding site for cross-bridging (hydrolysis of ATP to ADP + P via the ATPase enzymic process).

2. On the myosin filament to cause it to detach from actin following the cross-bridge power stroke.

3. At the site that transports Ca+ and K in and out of the fiber to and from the sarcoplasmic reticulum (SR).

Go to this link to view a live animation of the endpoint of contraction at the molecular level. It is quite fascinating to see the various chemicals moving about their business to fulfill their role in the cross-bridging process: *http://www.sci.sdsu.edu/movies/actin_myosin_gif.html* (17)

— So, Here's What's Important to Know —

1. At the molecular level a single muscle contraction involves a coordinated effort among many chemicals and substructures.

2. Sodium (Na), Potassium (K), Calcium (Ca), Magnesium (Mg), and the energy molecule Adenosine Triphosphate (ATP) are all involved in the contraction process.

3. A lack of ATP will prevent the actin-myosin filament cross-bridging and thus will shut down muscle contraction.

4

ENERGY SYSTEMS FUELING MUSCLE

The CNS signal-sending, chemical-structural interacting, and resultant force output actions (dynamic or static) are fascinating. And that all-important ATP molecule essentially being the energy substrate that fuels all contractions. What about the energy needed for not only single muscle contractions, but for long-term, extended events such as high reps and multiple sets?

Prior to discussing that, it is prudent to gain a basic understanding of the body's energy systems. Although much of it goes beyond the scope of resistance training, it is important to understand the entire spectrum of energy for muscle contraction using other activities. Consider these energy requirements:

- Low force needed for long periods of time (i.e., running 40 minutes).

- High force needed for short periods of time (i.e., offensive lineman drive blocking a defender).

- A combination of varied low, moderate, and high forces needed over various periods of time (i.e., an athletic contest where various low to high forces from one to 15 seconds each occur in an entire 15 to 90-minute period, such as a basketball game or tennis match).

Whatever the amount of force and length of time required, that cell energy molecule ATP must be available to fuel it. This is where the body's energy systems manufacture ATP, and it can be supplied three ways depending on the intensity of effort required: 1) ATP-PC system, 2) glycolysis, and 3) aerobic respiration.

1. **ATP-PC.** Immediate stores in the muscle up to :03, then :12 to :15 of additional time from stored creatine phosphate (CP) via the creatine kinase (CK) reaction which quickly replenishes

ATP: ATP ➡ energy + ADP, then CP + ADP = new ATP for immediate use. Assuring an adequate supply of stored creatine phosphate allows for those extra few seconds of maximal effort.

Examples: A heavy set of four reps in a resistance exercise or a 100-meter sprint.

NOTE: Assuring an adequate supply of intramuscular creatine stores – either through dietary intake or creatine supplementation – can extend maximum effort a few seconds. The extra molecules of creatine phosphate (CP) augment the creatine kinase (CK) reaction where a phosphate (P) is added to ADP (from the hydrolysis of an ATP molecule) to form new ATP.

---

2. **GLYCOLYSIS.** Beyond :15 up to 1:30 through glycolysis via the breakdown of glucose (sugar). This glucose can come from its circulation in the blood stream, from its storage as glycogen in the muscles, and/or from the liver via the process of glyco-genolysis (breakdown of glycogen to glucose).

   Examples: A moderately heavy set of 15 to 25 reps in a resistance exercise or a 400-meter run.

   Both the ATP-PC system and glycolysis provide ATP for muscle contraction without inhaling oxygen; hence they are anaerobic. However, their potential to supply ATP is limited which explains why high effort/high force work cannot be sustained for long periods.

3. **AEROBIC.** The third means of supplying ATP is aerobically via inhaled oxygen. The aerobic respiration system is virtually endless in the amount of ATP it can supply, but it takes time to completely "kick in" due to the time of its processing through the mitochondria (at least 2:00 for full activation).

   Examples: Using a resistance training example to describe the aerobic system is not practical, but a light set performed for an ultra-high number of reps or time (i.e., 60+ reps/3:00+). A more practical example would be a 10K run.

   Although there are many factors affecting a person's overall ability — muscle fiber type, body fat percentage, skeletal lever-age, and training status (trained or untrained) to name a few —

consider energy supply by itself: imagine if one executed an all-out sprint to chase someone. At approximately :30 into that venture they would begin to experience muscle discomfort due to the rapid production of ATP from the two anaerobic systems, and consequently an increase in metabolite accumulation. From that point their running speed would begin to decline. They could continue running hard, albeit at a slower speed, and around the 1:00 point even further slowing would ensue. Around the 1:30 point they would be feeling like a week-old TV dinner, moving much slower, but still able to move. Beyond that point their aerobic "I need oxygen" system that had been slowing revving up is finally able to generate ATP and their ability to recover from the prior high effort can occur.

In the beginning they could move fast, relying on the ATP-PC and glycolysis systems. Because those systems are high power but quicker to fatigue their speed declined as the slower-to-assist aerobic system was only contributing minimally. Relying solely on oxygen to generate ATP takes longer, but a few minutes into that slower speed mode allows for some recovery of the anaerobic systems. If they then attempted to pick up the speed and rely on the anaerobic systems again, their ability would depend on their level of conditioning.

It is important to know all three energy systems overlap, but it is the intensity of effort which determines which one is mostly relied upon. In resistance training, heavier, low-rep sets rely on mostly on the ATP-PC system for immediate ATP production. As reps progress up to double digits, glycolysis becomes more important. Sets performed for a high number of reps are still primarily glycolysis events, but the aerobic system slowly becomes a contributor, especially when a set is performed for those ultra-high reps that exceed 2:00.

Whatever the case, possessing better overall strength and endurance via a well-balanced training program will improve the ability to lift heavier resistance and perform more repetitions with relative submaximal resistances, all other factors being equal (more on this in the Training Status and Nutrition section).

— So, Here's What's Important to Know —

1. Muscles need the molecule ATP to contract. ATP can be generated from A) immediate stores and the creatine kinase reaction via stored creatine phosphate (:00 to :15), B) glycolysis via

glucose and stored glycogen (:15 to 1:30), and C) aerobically via oxygen intake (over 2:00).

2. All three energy systems are available at the outset of an activity, but the intensity of effort dictates which one is relied upon the most. Immediate ATP stores are there for short term high effort demands. As the activity continues, glycolysis and oxygen intake become more important to produce ATP. At any given point of any activity – from short term/high intensity to long term/low intensity – the sum product of ATP generated by all energy systems equals 100%.

3. It is mostly an ATP-PC and glycolysis discussion when it comes to resistance training due to most programs prescribing reps under 30-ish. The "30-ish" prescribed repetitions may take up to 1:30 to complete (depending on the rep execution velocity and cadence) which falls within the glycolysis time frame. However, there is value in performing ultra-high reps (60+/ 3:00) which will be discussed later.

4. When it comes to one's MU/fiber type make up and ATP availability, much of it comes down to the amount of resistance used and the number of reps performed. That is, those with an above average quantity of type 2X MUs/fibers, average 2A, and below average type 1 (less endurance potential) may possess a heavier 1-RM than a person with an average quantity of type 1, above average 2A, and below average type 2X (more endurance potential). Other factors must be considered (i.e., training status and neurological ability), but when it comes to maximum reps performed to MMF with a submaximal resistance (i.e., 75% of their own 1-RM), the latter more enduring but weaker person may be able to perform more reps with that amount of resistance compared to the less enduring but stronger person.

5. Creatine intake via one's diet and/or supplementation can extend maximum efforts for a few additional seconds due to a maximal supply of phosphocreatine needed to resynthesize ATP in the CK reaction.

6. Performing progressive resistance training over a period of weeks improves ATP supply and enhances muscle force capacity. Consequently, both the ability to A) lift relatively heavier resistances and B) perform more repetitions with sub-maximum resistances increase compared to one's prior untrained state.

5

CAUSES OF FATIGUE

Any physical event when pushed to the limit will result in some type of fatigue and, consequently, a decrease in performance whether it is a short-term resistance training set or a long-term endurance event like a marathon run.

Muscle fatigue – the inability to produce force at the required level – is caused by numerous factors. Aside from the soon-to-be-discussed training status and nutritional intake (and to some extent one's type 1 vs. type 2 MU/fiber type and quantity), fatigue occurs because of two issues:

1. **Central fatigue (CNS)**. From the brain through the motor neurons to the motor end plate, central fatigue occurs due to compromises in the CNS that decrease voluntary muscle contraction. The central fatigue-causing factors include the following (18):

   - A decrease of the stimulus to the motor neuron (MN).

   - Increased inhibition input to the MN due to afferent feedback from sensory cells.

   - Impairment of the MN itself.

   Central fatigue in resistance training is usually an issue when it comes to training volume. Within a training session the performance of mega-multiple sets per muscle group (i.e., 8+) can lead to central fatigue. This is particularly true when one performs high reps to fatigue (i.e., 20+). In addition, total weekly training volume can also create central fatigue if the recovery time between training sessions is inadequate.

2. **Peripheral fatigue**. Inside muscle is where peripheral fatigue occurs. This is the type of fatigue which most think of when discussing fatigue.

Peripheral fatigue entails impairment of mechanisms from the excitation/coupling process to the cross-bridging actin and myosin due to (19):

- An increase in muscle acidity; metabolite accumulation depending on the fate of pyruvate to either lactate or lactic acid.

- A decrease in available ATP at required sites.

- A disruption of calcium movement, either depletion or excessive accumulation.

Specifically, there is a difference between type 1 and the type 2 MUs/fibers depending on the workload they experience. In higher rep sets performed to MMF, the excitation/coupling contraction ability of the more enduring but lower force generating type 1 MUs/fibers can be impaired, but they do not truly reach complete failure. On the other hand, both type 2 MUs/fibers (because they are less fatigue resistant) are the reason further reps cannot be performed independent of the number of reps performed to MMF. They are affected more by the three factors that impair the excitation/coupling and actin/myosin cross-bridging mechanisms.

Related to that is the reality of one's MU/fiber type quantity and distribution in the muscles performing an exercise. All other factors being equal, if one possesses an above average quantity of type 2X MUs/fibers they will fatigue sooner (complete fewer reps) in relatively heavy sets in the 10 to 20 rep range as compared to one with an above average quantity of type 2A MUs/fibers. However, the former will be able to use a comparatively heavier resistance than the latter.

Peripheral fatigue in resistance training is always a consideration when establishing any resistance training program due to more short-term issues. Depending on one's training goal, each set performed requires appropriate recovery time between sets. This is due to the complex interaction between minerals, ATP availability, the extent of muscle acidity, and if complete recovery or only partial recovery is desired relative to that training goal (i.e., pure strength or a conditioning effect).

In general, to effectively perform low rep/heavy resistance sets more rest between sets is needed. If performing high rep/light resistance sets as a means of elevating the heart rate (i.e., circuit-type workouts) then naturally less rest time between sets would be prudent.

Knowing the specific cause(s) of fatigue can facilitate better training program design regarding not only specific exercise sets and reps, but also the scheduling of training days. That will assure the complete recovery of all central or peripheral fatigue factors.

— So, Here's What's Important to Know —

1. Muscle fatigue results from many factors. Regardless, the inability to produce the required force to continue performing reps is a byproduct of one or more issues occurring from the motor cortex in the brain to the chemical interactions required for actin and myosin to crossbridge and produce muscle contraction.

2. Central fatigue involves impairments in the CNS from the motor cortex in the brain to the muscle. Peripheral fatigue involves disruption of events inside the muscle fibers, mainly the accumulation and/or unavailability of chemical substrates involved with actin and myosin cross-bridging.

3. Naturally, possessing more faster-to-fatigue type 2X MUs/fibers will lead to quicker fatigue as compared to possessing more type 2A MUs/fibers. The possession of more or less type 1 would also factor into potential results depending on the proportion of the other two, all other factors being equal.

4. Understanding the causes of fatigue will facilitate better training program design regarding the proper dosage of sets, reps, and total training volume during single workout sessions and multiple sessions over the training period. That will assure adequate recovery and adaptation to compliment reasonable progressive training over the long term.

6

OTHER GENETIC FACTORS

Genetic make-up has a significant influence on one's ability to execute a resistance training set. Ironically, it is often-times overlooked when it comes to performance expectations and setting realistic goals. Not to discount hard work, training consistency, and mental focus, the unalterable genetic factors largely determine one's potential to display muscle force output in various situations.

Aside from the previous discussions on the genetic factors of body type (endo-, meso-, and ectomorph), inherent quantity of the three MUs/fiber types, and their between muscle differences, other genetic factors must be considered when assessing the outcomes of various resistance training sets. This would include the following:

1. **Skeletal leverage:** the configuration of bone length, tendon insertions, and muscle belly length at all skeletal joints in the involved exercise (see figures 7, 8, 9, and 10 below).

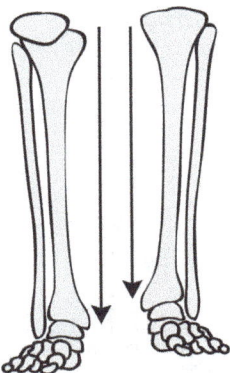

Figure 7: Length of the Bones in the Skeletal System

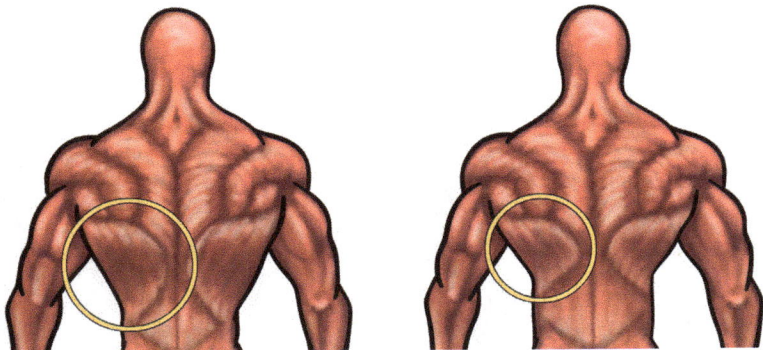

Figure 8: Muscle Belly Length – left: longer muscle belly; right: shorter muscle belly

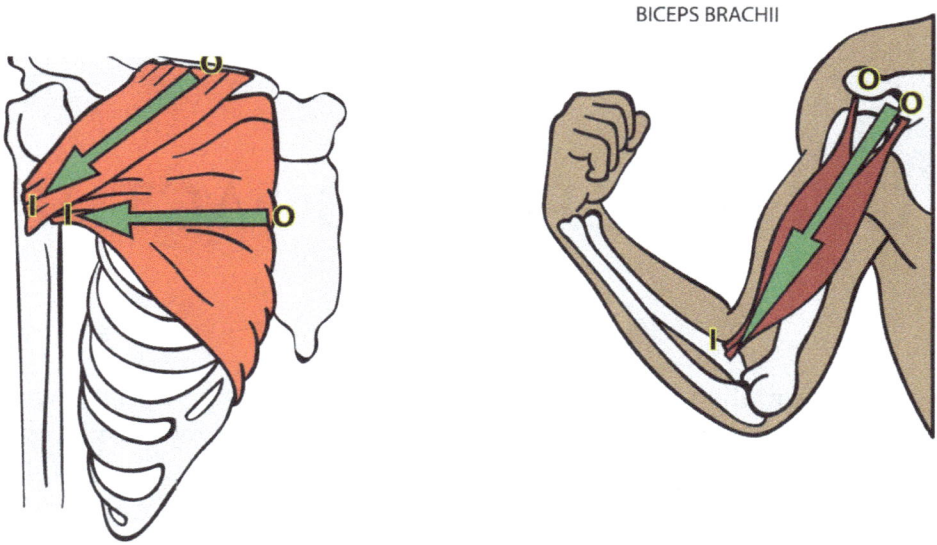

BICEPS BRACHII

Figure 9: Tendon Insertion (I) and origins (O) on the Skeletal System

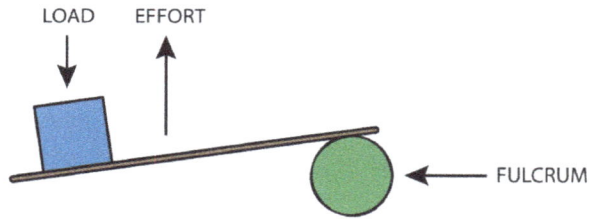

LOAD   EFFORT

FULCRUM

Figure 10: Third Class Lever (above); Combined Bone Length and Tendon Insertion Point Leverage (below)

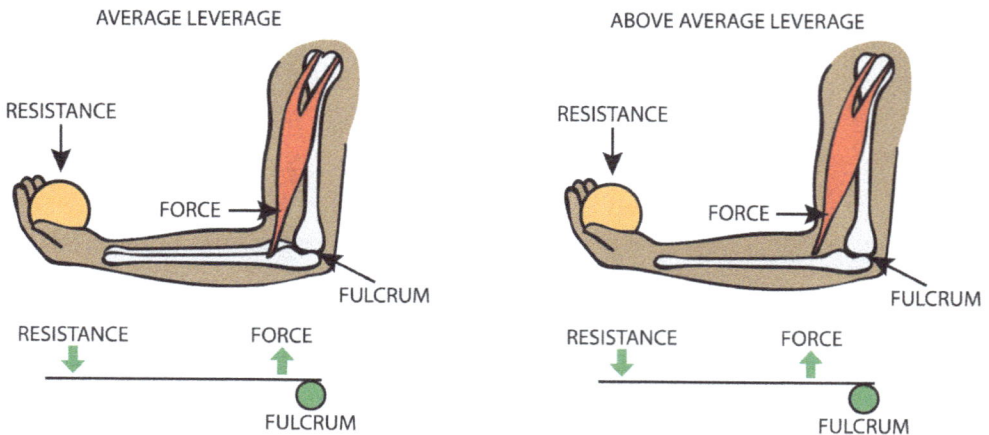

AVERAGE LEVERAGE

RESISTANCE

FORCE

FULCRUM

RESISTANCE   FORCE

FULCRUM

ABOVE AVERAGE LEVERAGE

RESISTANCE

FORCE

FULCRUM

RESISTANCE   FORCE

FULCRUM

All other factors being equal, the following skeletal leverage factors create a *mechanical advantage* when resistance training:

- Shorter bones (levers) as compared to longer bones (figure 7).

- Shorter muscle bellies as compared to longer bellies (figure 8).

- More favorable tendon insertion points on the skeleton (figure 9) relative to the resistance, force (pull), and fulcrum (pivot point) at the relevant joint(s) (figure 10) in accordance with the class 3 lever.

But it is not always at one joint as in the above figures. Multi-joint resistance exercises such as chest and shoulder presses, pulldowns and rows, and squatting, dead lifting, and leg pressing require multiple muscle groups acting on more than one skeletal joint. Therefore, the entire dynamic of the specific exercise relative to each joint and its structure adds another level of consideration. Various combinations of below average, average, and above average joint configurations exist and affect performance potential.

2. **Neurological ability/CNS potential**: Regarding the 70% rule where it is impossible to recruit all MUs/fibers at one time, there can be genetic differences between people regarding how many can potentially be activated. The 70% rule is approximate and can be used as the average when it comes to most discussions and comparisons. However, in some cases there may be people who can recruit more than 70% and some less than 70%. This phenomenon was introduced to the strength training world by the late Arthur Jones, founder of Nautilus Sports Medical Industries in the 1970s. Arthur was a man way ahead of his time and was often caustic and biting in his demeanor. He labeled the CNS potential-to-recruit MUs/fibers as Neurological Ability (NA). To this day minimal research has been applied to it, but it is worthy of discussion because some people can exhibit odd outcomes due to it.

   Any forthcoming discussion and speculation on NA (referred to as NA/CNS potential from this point forward) will be presented in respect to its likely existence and the need to consider it.

It's possible for one person to possess an above average NA/CNS potential (i.e., 73%) while another a below average NA/CNS potential (i.e., 65%). In simple terms, if three people possessed 500 MUs in the same muscle, the average person would be able to recruit 350 (70% of 500), the above average 365 (73% of 500), and the below average 325 (65% of 500).

Understandably, differences in NA/CNS potential may have a significant impact on the amount of resistance they can lift in a 1-RM and likewise in submaximal resistance sets for multiple reps. It is still contingent on the type and quantity of MUs/fibers and other genetic factors, but all other factors being equal, one with an above average NA/CNS potential will be able to produce a higher 1-RM as compared to one possessing an average or below average NA/CNS potential.

Regarding the reserve pool discussion and submaximal resistance/multiple rep sets to MMF, the situations and outcomes can vary regarding both above and below average NA/CNS potential. Understand that a person only recruits the minimum number of MUs/fibers to complete each rep relative to 1) the amount of resistance used, 2) their NA/CNS potential, and 3) their MU/fiber type quantity and distribution. But the ability to recruit an above average of all types means more MUs/fibers will be involved each rep (with a relatively heavier amount of resistance), fewer will therefore be in reserve, thus a lesser number of reps can be performed. On that, possessing more type 1 and 2A MUs/fibers will at the least allow for the completion of more reps in very high rep sets as compared to someone who possess fewer of those but a greater quantity of the faster-to-fatigue 2X MUs/fibers.

Comparatively, possessing a below average NA/CNS potential goes the opposite way: The person is weaker due to the inability to recruit many MUs/fibers each rep, but that will allow for a greater reserve pool of unrecruited MUs/fibers which can extend the set for more reps, albeit with a lighter relative resistance.

The point to understand is one may be stronger due in part to an above average NA/CNS potential, but their ability to perform multiple reps with a submaximal resistance is diminished, relatively speaking. Similarly, a below average NA/CNS – all other factors being equal – equates to a lower 1-RM, but more potential to complete a greater number of reps with the same percentage of a their 1-RM (but with a lighter resistance).

This topic will be further discussed in detail regarding various potential outcomes between people relative to 1) the reps achieved in submaximal resistance sets, 2) the amount of resistance used in those sets relative to not only their 1-RM but also their NA/CNS potential, and 3) their inherent MU/fiber type quantity and distribution throughout the acting muscle groups.

3. **The reality of all genetic factors combined:** Different genetic abilities can be depicted using the normal distribution curves to better see the reality of combined traits and the wide variety of possibilities. The normal curve presentation of genetic differences is used in context to simply show differences to better see why there are the rare exceptionally talented world-class athletes on one end and genetic trash bag weekend warriors on the other.

    Figure 11 below depicts different body types and muscle mass volumes. An average person (male or female) would reside in the green segment. The hypothetical exceptions – more obese on the left and more muscular/lean on the right – would fall in the 13.59% segments and beyond.

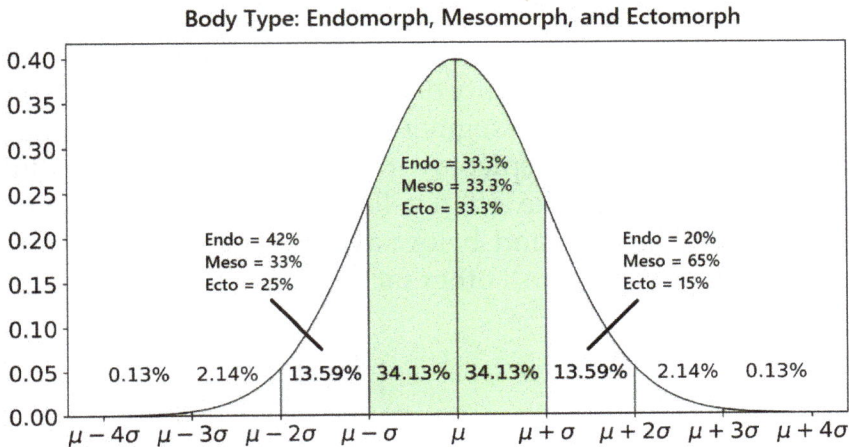

Figure 11: Body Type

Regarding skeletal leverage (combination of bone length, muscle belly size, and tendon insertions), many possible combinations can exist. Whatever "average" would be regarding skeletal configurations, the average person would reside in the red segment of figure 12. The hypothetical below average on the left would depict disadvantageous long levers and poor tendon insertions in terms of exhibiting pure strength as an example. The above average on the right would be the opposite: short levers and advantageous muscle insertions which would facilitate greater strength. Whatever skeletal leverage combinations one possesses, they would fall somewhere on the curve that distributes all possible skeletal leverage differences.

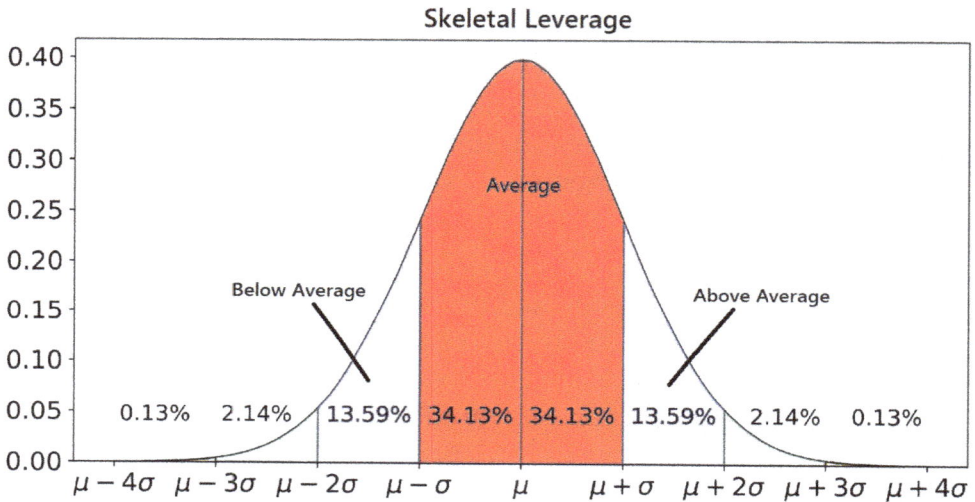

Figure 12: Skeletal Leverage

Regarding MU/fiber type quantity, one could possess a favorable-for-strength above average quantity of 2X, average 2A, and below average type 1 as depicted in the blue segment on the right in figure 13. If the normal curve were used to depict favorable-for-local muscle endurance potential, the depiction on the left in yellow with an average quantity of type 1, above average 2A, and below average 2X MUs/fibers would have the advantage for that, all other factors being equal.

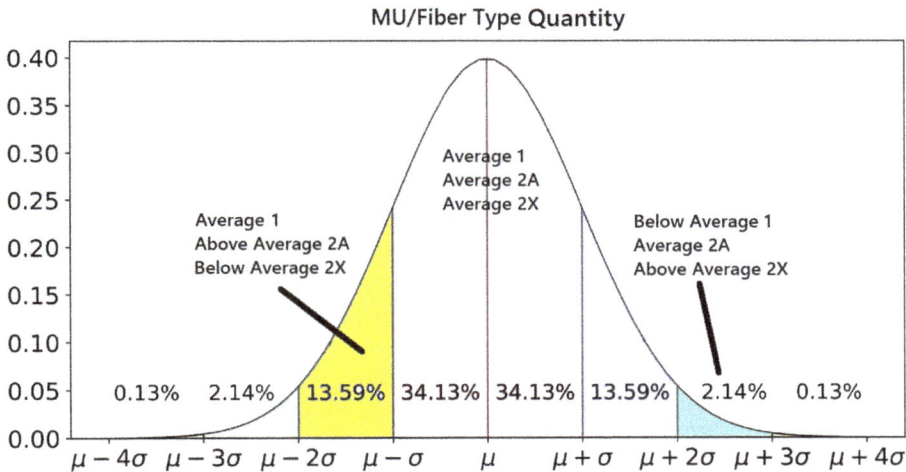

Figure 13: MU/Fiber Type Quantity (favorable for strength)

Regarding MU/fiber type distribution between three acting muscle groups during an exercise, one could possess the more-favorable-for-strength combinations in the 13.59% green segment on the right in figure 14.

Using a bench press as an example, muscle A would be the pectorals, B the anterior deltoids, and C the triceps:

- Muscle A pectorals @ **below average** quantity of type 1, **above average** 2A, and average 2X.
- Muscle B anterior deltoids @ average quantity of each type.
- Muscle C triceps @ **below average** quantity of type 1, average 2A, and **above average** 2X.

All combined, they would possess a **slight above average** quantity of the strongest 2X (average-average-**above average**) and a **slight above average** quantity of the stronger-than-type 1 2A (**above average**-average-average). Their strength potential in the bench press would therefore be above average.

In comparison, the white 13.59% section on the left would be less-favorable-for-strength as follows:

- Muscle A pectorals @ average quantity of each type.
- Muscle B anterior deltoids @ **above average** type 1, average 2A, and **below average** 2X.

- Muscle C triceps @ average type 1, **above average** 2A, and **below average** 2X.

MU/Fiber Type Distribution Between Three Acting Muscle Groups
(in order: Type 1, 2A, and 2X)

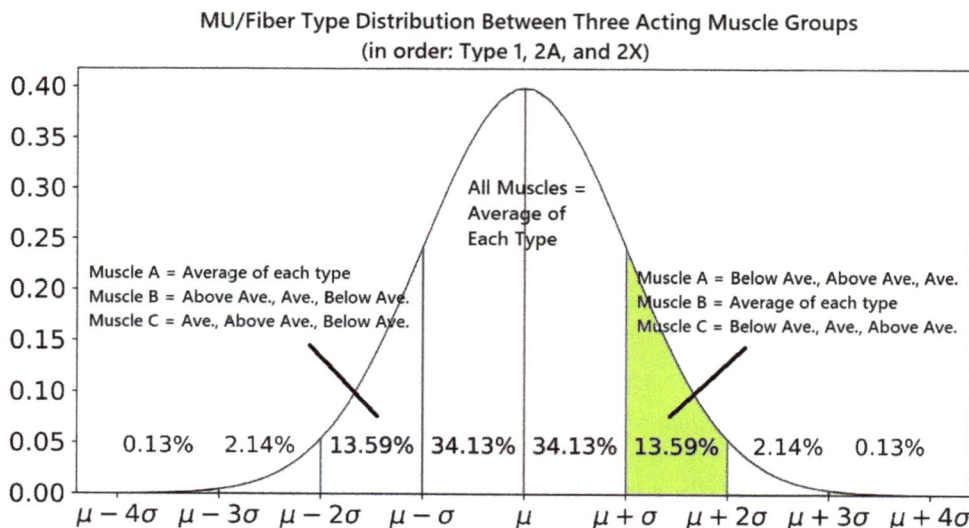

Figure 14: MU/Fiber Type Distribution

Regarding NA/CNS potential, one could be 70% (average), 73% (above average), or 67% (below average). As depicted in the purple segment on the left in figure 15, the below average ability to contract a maximum number of MUs/fibers in a single effort would indicate a relative low strength ability, all other factors being equal.

Understand the figure below reflects maximum strength potential, but similar to the hypothetical example of MU/fiber type distribution in figure 14, that below average NA/CNS potential person would possess greater relative ability in local muscle endurance due to a greater reserve pool from which to extend the number of reps performed with sub-maximal resistances as compared to an average or above average NA/CNS potential.

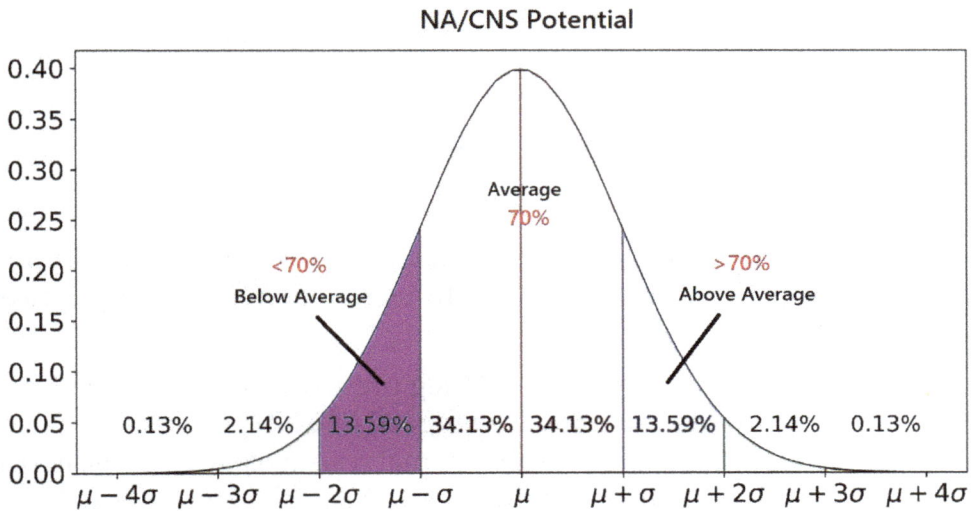

Figure 15: NA/CNS Potential for Strength

COMBINING MU/FIBER TYPE QUANTITY AND NA/CNS POTENTIAL

Making distinctions among the population by comparing all characteristics and abilities can be even more confounding when combining both NA/CNS potential and MU/fiber type quantity and distribution to the mix.

Using a 1-RM leg press exercise as an example (maximum strength expression as opposed to local muscle endurance), if two people have 600 MUs controlling 900,000 muscle fibers in their quadriceps, it may look like this (remember, the total quantity of MUs/fibers must equal 600/900,000 in some combination of below average, average, and above average):

Average would be considered this:

– Type 1: 300 MUs/450,000 fibers.

– Type 2A: 210 MUs/315,000 fibers.

– Type 2X: 90 MUs/135,000 fibers.

Person 1

– The average quantity of all types as noted above.

  • + an above average NA/CNS potential.

Person 2

- Below average quantity of type 1 (240 MUs/360,000 fibers).

- Above average type 2A (270/405,000).

- Average type 2X (90/135,000).

- + an average NA/CNS potential.

What would be their potentials regarding 1-RM leg press ability and the maximum number of reps to MMF using submaximal resistances based on the 1-RMs?

Person 1 = an above average 1-RM leg press due to an average MU/fiber type make up plus an above average NA/CNS potential? A fewer number of reps performed with submaximal resistances due to the above average NA/CNS potential and thus fewer MU/fibers in reserve?

Person 2 = A slight above average 1-RM leg press due to an average NA/CNS potential, but a combined above average quantity of both type 2A and 2X MUs/fibers? A slight above average ability to perform more reps in the leg press due to the above average quantity of the slightly-weaker-than-type 2X but more enduring intermediate 2A MUs/fibers?

COMBINED MU/FIBER TYPE QUANTITY & NA/CNS POTENTIAL ON THE NORMAL DISTRIBUTION CURVE: POSSIBLE COMBINATIONS REGARDING 1-RM STRENGTH POTENTIAL

Centerline of curve

Average 1-RM strength potential.

Example: All MUs/fiber type quantities and NA/CNS potential are average.

Right side 34.13% section

Slight above average for a greater 1-RM.

Example: below average type 1, above average 2A, and average 2X + an average NA/CNS potential.

Left side 34.13% section

Slight below average for a lesser 1-RM.

Example: above average type 1, below average 2A, and average 2X + an average NA/CNS potential.

Right side 13.59% section

Above average for a greater 1-RM.

Example: below average type 1, average 2A, and above average 2X + an average NA/CNS potential.

Left side 13.59% section

Below average for a lesser 1-RM.

Example: above average type 1, average 2A, and below average 2X + an average NA/CNS potential.

Right side 2.14% section

Way above average for a much greater 1-RM.

Example: below average type 1, average 2A, and above average 2X + above average NA/CNS potential.

Left side 2.14% section

Way below average for a much lesser 1-RM.

Example: above average type 1, average 2A, and below average 2X + below average NA/CNS potential.

Right side 0.13% section

Superior ability for a world class 1-RM.

Example: way below average type 1, average 2A, and way above average 2X + way above average NA/CNS potential.

Left side 0.13% section

Inferior ability for a genetic trash bag 1-RM.

Example: way above average type 1, average 2A, and way below average 2X + way below average NA/CNS potential.

COMBINING ALL GENETIC FACTORS

Using all distribution curve examples from figures 11 through 15, transpose the body type curve (fig. 11) example (average) on the skeletal leverage curve (fig. 12) (average) and you begin to see one possible combination. Add the favorable-for-strength MU/fiber quantity curve (fig. 13) and it further becomes unique. Finally, transpose both the favorable-for-strength MU/fiber distribution curve (green segment, fig. 14) and the below average NA/CNS potential curve (purple segment, fig. 15) on the others and the diversity continues. Literally hundreds of combinations exist.

Think of those freaky people who can demonstrate exceptional abilities in not only strength and endurance expressions in resistance exercise bouts, but also in running speed, ultra endurance contests, and explosive events. They may possess a favorable body type, a large quantity and favorable distribution of relevant MUs/fibers, exceptional skeletal leverage, and an ideal NA/CNS potential for their respective sport. Conversely, you have the opposite end of the spectrum that includes horrible performers who can't get out of their own way and have the speed of a turtle on crutches in molasses going backward; essentially unfavorable genetics all around.

— So, Here's What's Important to Know —

1. Genetic make-up significantly impacts the potential in the amount of resistance one can use in a resistance training exercise as well as the ability to run fast, jump high, hit hard, and throw far, to name a few.

2. The genetic factors of body type (and relative muscle mass), skeletal leverage, MU/fiber type quantity, their between-muscle groups distribution of MUs/fibers, and one's NA/CNS potential all must be considered. Their effect on performance potential can vary from minimal to extreme.

3. Many combinations of the genetic factors exist among the population. There are literally hundreds of possibilities that involve below average, average, and above average characteristics. That results in a wide range of abilities from horribly unfavorable/poor to exceptionally favorable/excellent.

4. Most genetic factors are unalterable but through intelligent and progressive training anyone can maximize their potential.

7

TRAINING STATUS AND NUTRITION

Training on a regular basis using some form of progressive training and complimenting that with reasonable nutritional intake will maximize one's genetic potential regardless of physical endowment.

A person will have more potential to exhibit greater effort in any force exertion event if they have 1) used some system of increasing the workload in terms of an increased amount of resistance and/or number of reps performed and 2) consumed a reasonable type and amount of food as compared to:

1. Their previous untrained state.

2. Their previous poor nutritional intake state.

3. Someone with less genetic potential.

4. Someone with the same genetic potential but is untrained and/ or has poor nutritional habits.

5. In some cases someone with better genetic potential but is untrained and/or has poor nutritional habits.

Regarding progressive training, over the course of a multi-week training plan one learns how to recruit more MUs/fibers, forces those MUs/fibers to grow and adapt to training stresses, and consequently improves muscle force output capacity.

Regarding nutrition, its effect on resistance training centers on 1) possessing enough energy substrate to fuel the performance of exercise sets, 2) post-workout energy replenishment, and 3) protein intake to facilitate muscle repair and growth.

Remember, ATP and minerals are required for a muscle to contract. They ultimately are derived from the intake of the macronutrients carbohydrates (carbs), fats, and proteins (proteins only in unique situations). The average person's dietary intake provides enough energy for immediate ATP stores, ATP circulating in the blood via glucose stored in the liver and muscles (glycogen), and ATP stored in the adipose fat sites (triglycerides). This is due mostly to the high amount of carbs most consume in a standard diet.

Rather than go into the intricate details of macronutrient breakdown, storage, and use for energy, just know this: an over-abundance of quick-digesting simple carbs in addition to slower-to-digest complex carbs consumed daily will provide those immediate, circulating, and stored energy forms. Unless one is hard-core fasting and not eating for days, adequate energy to fuel resistance training workouts should be available for most people. Even if one goes into Ketosis by drastically reducing total carb intake, Ketone bodies will be produced which supplant carbs as an alternative energy source. Therefore, not having at least a minimum amount of ATP available is rarely an issue in resistance training, but it could be an issue during ultra-endurance competitions when energy is needed for lengthy periods (i.e., consumption of quick digesting carbs and/or carb supplements during an Ironman competition).

Regarding protein intake, most registered dieticians recommend .8 grams per kilogram (2.2 pounds) of body weight as a daily minimum (20). However, it is common for many to fail to ingest an adequate amount to build and repair muscle. When resistance training it's safe to ingest at least .8 to 1.0 gram of protein per pound (.454 kilograms) of body weight. It is better to go a bit over than sadly not consume enough of it.

The human body is in constant flux, so to maintain an ideal nitrogen balance protein consumption should occur throughout the day aiming for intake every three to four hours. However, the reason why many trainees fail to ingest enough daily is due to the reliance solely on the traditional three-feeding times: breakfast, lunch, and dinner. If one is a traditional three meals/day creature of habit simply plan a between-meal protein intake that will more easily allow for the .8 to 1.0 gram/pound goal. That can be accomplished by consuming healthy protein-rich food options available from the local supermarket and many easy-to-consume reputable protein supplement options.

— So, Here's What's Important to Know —

1. Training intelligently and progressively will maximize one's genetic potential and allow them to exhibit greater resistance training force outputs as compared to their previous untrained state and/or poor nutritional intake status.

2. Likewise, doing the above may improve one's ability to out-perform another person with equal ability, or in some cases out-perform a person who possess better genetics but who is un-trained and poorly nourished.

3. The average person's diet is usually able to supply food intake-generated ATP and the pertinent minerals for A) both high force/low rep and low force/high rep resistance training sets and B) the between training session replenishment of muscle and liver glycogen stores.

4. Consuming an appropriate amount of protein daily will posi-tively affect the potential for muscle to repair itself and grow larger. Focus on .8 to 1.0 gram per pound (.454 kg) of body weight. Use feeding sessions every three to four hours to facili-tate reaching the daily goal.

8

SKILLS ACQUISITION AND ENHANCEMENT

In general, there are two types of skills when it comes to athletic performance: open skills and closed skills.

Closed skills involve fewer factors that affect performance. This would include most resistance training exercises. In closed skills there is an exact starting point and ending point of the task to be completed, such as a push up, dumbbell squat, or seated row.

Open skills involve more performance-affecting factors, such as moving in various directions, performing an assortment of intra-sport skill requirements, and dealing with the unpredictability of opponents. Open skills would include such sports as tennis, football, or ice hockey, to name a few.

Both open and closed skill practice, acquisition, and enhancement should be based on the Principle of Specificity. The basic tenet of the Principle of Specificity is straight-forward: to become better at something the exact practice of whatever that something is must be the focus. Not almost. Not close to. Not sort of. It's exact replication over and over. Whether it's a specific individual skill or series of contingency-based skill sets, one must repeatedly practice them exactly as they will be required during a contest.

The principle of specificity has been misunderstood for decades. The reasons are simple: 1) few have taken the time to study the proven research on skill specificity and 2) there is money to be made off well-intended but ignorant seekers of improved skills. That is a long discussion and beyond the scope of this segment, so here is how the specificity principle applies to resistance training.

Being a closed skill, the great majority of resistance training exercises are easy to master with repeated practice. Awkward at first, but more proficient as time is spent repeating them over and over.

Most people have experienced this when they first started "lifting" on a regular basis, whether it was a barbell bench press, barbell squat, plate-load leg press, or even that power clean the high school football coach made mandatory: When first attempting the exercise, it was unfamiliar and awkward. There was a need to use relatively lighter resistance as well. There was also that inevitable muscle soreness that appeared and lasted for days following the first session. Over time as the exercise was performed on a continual basis for weeks and months in scheduled training sessions, they were then able to move the resistance with better technique, progressively increase the amount of resistance used, and muscle soreness diminished following each successive training session. The specific skills of proper exercise performance improved due to better intramuscular coordination, repeated practice of the movement, and the ability to progressively recruit more MUs/fibers within their inherent NA/CNS potential.

On that, note these points:

1. Becoming stronger in the pectorals and triceps by using a machine-type chest press and single joint tricep exercise, for example, will improve the ability to lift more resistance in a barbell bench press, but not as much as regularly using the barbell bench press itself to maximally improve ability in that exercise. Remember: specificity is all about exactness.

2. Likewise, many devices and exercises can be used to improve the force capacity of a specific muscle or combination of muscle groups. In example, to target the upper back muscles one can use wide and narrow grip chin ups, wide and narrow grip plate-load or selectorized machine pulldowns, or any seated, bent-over, or low row. They all engage those muscles but with different modes or devices. All can be effective provided they are performed with proper technique and create an overload stress on those muscles. Like moving from point A to B in an automobile; it can be done in a 1973 Mercury Capri, 1982 Ford Mustang II, or a 2010 Jeep Patriot. They all work if one drives them properly.

3. Increasing muscle strength using naturally slower moving and relatively heavier resistances will improve one's power (force x distance/time) and thus the ability to move lighter resistance at a faster velocity, all other factors being equal. In example, performing relatively slow-moving heavy dead lifts, elbow

flexion exercises (bicep curls), and exercises that target the deltoids and trapezius (upright rows) will improve the potential to perform Olympic-style lifts (i.e., cleans, snatches, and their variations) with greater resistances provided the skills of the Olympic lifts are also practiced concurrently (again, the exactness of specificity).

— SO, HERE'S WHAT'S IMPORTANT TO KNOW —

1. In resistance training – a closed skill – one will improve on any exercise by virtue of performing it on a regular basis (essentially, practicing it exactly).

2. Once one masters the skill of an exercise, further strength and size improvements occur from 1) maximizing their NA/CNS potential within the neuromuscular system and 2) enhancing individual muscle fiber structural components in terms of strength and endurance.

3. Many modes and devices can be used to improve muscle force output potential provided they are used safely. To train the upper back and rear deltoids, for example, a barbell bent-over row, dumbbell 1-arm row, seated cable row, and plate-load machine low row can all be used. Any of those exercises can be used to create an overload stimulus on the acting muscle(s) provided they are performed regularly using a progressive set/ rep scheme each training session.

9

MOTIVATION AND MENTAL TOUGHNESS

This offers some hope for those genetically average or below average. If one has trained intelligently and progressively and has truly maxed out their genetic potential, they have a greater chance to out-perform someone of equal ability and possibly someone who possesses better ability if that person lacks motivation and/or is weak-minded.

A genetic freak with only a tincture of motivation and/or mental toughness can be defeated by a person with average genetics and a high level of motivation and mental toughness...in some instances. In team sports a group of highly motivated average abilities can defeat a group of superior abilities if the latter give a half-assed effort. It happens in all competitions and sports and I've seen it first-hand in the years I spent training athletes:

The underdog upsets the favorite team. They collectively find a way to out-perform the more talented opponent.

The specimen who had a "bad day" is defeated by the seemingly disadvantaged John or Jane Doe who exuded better mental toughness.

That supposed exceptional-ability person gives a poor effort because they think "Hey, I don't need to work hard" and they get their ass handed to them by a harder-working but less gifted person.

Now for the not-so-good news — that "in some instances" I mentioned. Regarding resistance training and possessing below average or even average genetics, especially the sports of powerlifting, weightlifting, and bodybuilding, if one is below average genetically (or even average in some cases), it is more difficult to out-perform someone with above average genetics. That is, they may never express the same strenth, muscle size, power, or physique compered to an above average genetic freak, especially if that more talented person is highly motivated and mentally tough.

Regarding workout sessions and maximizing one's potential: if a person is motivated to train hard and train consistently it will assure positive results, independent of genetic endowment. Being dedicated to a regularly performed progressive program – and having the mental toughness to push through demanding high intensity training sessions – will elevate anyone beyond another person of equal ability who lacks the motivation and drive to excel. That should be enough motivation for anyone to commit 100% compliance to working hard, eating properly and recovering properly.

One last item on motivation. Research has proven that motivation and encouragement via verbal commands by another poerson can increase force output (12). That is, trainees who are verbally encouraged prior to and during te performance of a resistance training set can exert greater effort. Therefore, it's okay if a trainer or training partner gets in your face and verbally steps it up a few notches to encourage effort, especially during excruciating high rep sets or gut-wrenching circuit-type workouts. Having someone insut your man- or womanhood is free, proven-to-work, and could make a big difference in results achieved.

— So, Here's What's Important to Know —

1. Genetic characteristics can affect the performance and results of resistance training exercises, both positively and negatively. It is difficult for an average or below average person to defeat a genetically above average person who is highly motivated to train hard and dedicated to all aspects of a resistance training program.

2. Regardless of genetic endowment, maximizing one's potential through a properly structured resistance training program and going all out when it counts will take anyone to their highest level of ability.

3. A competent trainer or training partner can offer additional verbal motivation to assure the trainee gives 100% effort in demanding sets performed.

10

PRACTICAL EXAMPLES

Finally. We are here. Getting to know the previous information – either the lengthy detailed sections or just the "So, Here's What's Important to Know" overviews – will help to understand the forthcoming resistance training set examples regarding the "What's going on in there" when muscles are called upon to complete them. Let's look at some examples and dissect them using the nine fundamentals of muscle contraction that were discussed.

DISCLAIMER: The forthcoming presentation is based on three things:

1. Proven research; facts.

2. Deductive reasoning; facts applied to subjective real-world examples.

3. Speculation; what is probably occurring – or close to it – based on the two prior points.

Someone needs to step forward and offer an interpretation of "What's going on in there" during a resistance training set. At least get the ball rolling so it can be critiqued and refined as research yet continues into the intricacies of muscle contraction in resistance training.

THE ANATOMY OF A 1-RM

EXERCISE EXAMPLE: BARBELL BENCH PRESS

ALL OTHER FACTORS BEING EQUAL...

MUSCLE FIBERS AND MOTOR UNITS (MUs)

The entire spectrum of MUs/fibers – types 1, 2A, and 2X – will be involved at their maximum recruitable role in the pectorals, anterior deltoid, and triceps to complete the 1-RM bench press.

Having a body type that has a greater volume of muscle in those muscles will increase the potential to lift more in a 1-RM attempt due to a greater volume of contractile tissue (see figure 2).

Specifically among the associated muscle groups, possessing an above average quantity of type 2X MU's/fibers in the involved pectorals, anterior deltoids, and/or triceps – even if one of those muscle groups is only average – would be more advantageous as compared to a person possessing only an average quantity and/or below average quantity in some combination.

THE NERVOUS SYSTEM

Through Henneman's Principle, a maximum recruitment of all recruitable MUs/fibers from type 1 through the larger and stronger type 2X - and within their specific NA/CNS potential - will be maximal from start to finish as it is an "all hands on deck" short term effort.

The rate coding (firing rate) will also be occurring at maximum. Through the type 1 ➡ type 2A ➡ type 2X order of recruitment each will be firing rapidly resulting in maximal cross-bridging of the fibers. A summation of force will create full tetanus in all MUs/fibers within the person's given NA/CNS potential. Because it is a heavy resistance moving at a slow bar velocity it is the epitome of maximum tension relative to the force-velocity curve, especially at the weakest point of the exercise range of motion (i.e., at the point of the range of motion where a second rep can not be completed).

A large reserve of MUs/fibers will remain at the completion of the event (all type 1, all type 2A, and approximately 65% of type 2X) due to the limited amount of time under tension. However, due to the fatigue of approximately 35% of the type 2X, the available reserve pool of MUs/fibers will be insufficient to perform a 2nd rep.

CHEMICAL INTERACTIONS AT THE MOLECULAR LEVEL

The presence of minerals calcium, magnesium, potassium, and sodium, and the energy molecule ATP (all originating from dietary intake) will facilitate the actin and myosin cross bridging and maximize muscle contraction during the 1-RM effort.

ENERGY SYSTEMS FUELING MUSCLE

The 1-RM is an event that takes only a few seconds to complete depending on the distance the bar must move from start to finish (see skeletal leverage discussion). It is primarily a stored ATP fueled event so the previous discussion on molecular level chemical interactions applies here as well.

CAUSES OF FATIGUE

The short nature of this 1-RM event is a result of a maximal number of all recruitable MUs/fibers creating the summation of force relative to one's NA/CNS potential. The immediate depletion of ATP in the higher threshold but low enduring 2X MUs/fibers (and the inability to fully replenish it) means that second rep cannot be performed. Thus, peripheral fatigue (even though minimal) will be the only fatigue factor due to the shortness of the 1-RM and lack of repetitive stress (as would be experienced in demanding multiple reps). Central fatigue will not be an issue.

OTHER GENETIC FACTORS

A favorable bone-tendon-muscle belly configuration will make it a mechanical advantage to lift a relatively heavier resistance in the 1-RM. This includes shorter arms, shorter muscle bellies, and above average tendon insertions on bones.

Possessing an above average NA/CNS potential (i.e., 74% of all) offers the ability to recruit an above average number of MUs/fibers in a maximal effort, thus a greater amount of resistance can be lifted. Couple that with an above average quantity of the strongest 2X MUs/fibers in the acting muscles and it would further increase one's 1-RM potential.

TRAINING STATUS AND NUTRITION

Regarding training, a person who has never resistance trained or has not performed it in a while (i.e., detrained) will improve their 1-RM bench press relative to their genetic potential provided they follow a relevant progressive training regimen.

Some possible examples:

	1-RM (pounds/kilograms)	
	DAY 1	**DAY 60**
Non-trained/below average genetics	150/68	175/80
Non-trained/average genetics	195/87	230/106
Trained/average genetics	215/98	240/109
Trained/above average genetics	305/139	330/150

As for nutrition, consuming a standard diet should supply the minerals and ATP substrate needed for a maximal 1-RM contraction in the associated bench-pressing muscle groups. If one has also consumed an adequate amount of protein over the course of the progressive training program used, it will facilitate muscle growth and repair which will also increase the potential to lift a heavier 1-RM.

SKILL ACQUISITION AND ENHANCEMENT

The bench press is a closed skill. Therefore, performing the bench press on a regular basis – including the periodic practice of performing a 1-RM – will optimize one's potential to lift the greatest amount of resistance possible within their genetic potential.

MOTIVATION AND MENTAL TOUGHNESS

Naturally, because the 1-RM is a brief maximal contraction, exuding 100% effort to recruit the maximum number of MUs/fibers to reach full tetanus within one's NA/CNS potential will enhance their potential to lift the greatest amount of resistance possible.

1-RM SUBJECT COMPARISONS

Regarding the MU/fiber quantity and distribution in each involved muscle group, ***the forthcoming hypotheticals note the quantity of type 2X only*** (most important for maximum strength due to their greater unit of force value) to better differentiate the abilities when comparing 1-RMs of eight subjects.

There are multiple possible combinations of all relevant genetic factors. Listed below are hypothetical subjects and their average and/or above average characteristics only. Obviously, the more above average one is, the greater their potential in a 1-RM.

> **NOTE:** In the following hypothetical examples, the categories of below average, average, and above average are somewhat subjective. But they reveal the variation between humans regarding all genetic factors. Therefore, a distinction must be made between abilities and characteristics which will help explain the various performance outcomes in resistance training.

FOUR FAVORABLE COMBINATIONS FOR DEMONSTRATING ABOVE AVERAGE STRENGTH:

Subject 1: 1-RM = 325 pounds/148 kilograms.

Average muscle volume.

Above average skeletal leverage.

MU/fiber type quantity and distribution:

- Average type 2X in the pectorals.

- **Above average** 2X in the deltoids.

- Average 2X in the triceps.

Above average NA/CNS potential.

Subject 2: 1-RM =315 pounds/143 kilograms.

Above average muscle volume.

Average skeletal leverage.

MU/fiber type quantity and distribution:

    – Average 2X in the pectorals.

    – Average 2X in the anterior deltoids.

    – **Above average** 2X in the triceps.

Above average NA/CNS potential.

Subject 3: 1-RM = 295 pounds/134 kilograms.

Average muscle volume.

Average skeletal leverage.

MU/fiber type quantity and distribution:

    – Average 2X in the pectorals.

    – Average 2X in the deltoids.

    – **Above average** 2X in the triceps.

Above average NA/CNS potential.

Subject 4: 1-RM = 360 pounds/164 kilograms.

Average muscle volume.

Above average skeletal leverage.

MU/fiber type quantity and distribution:

    – **Above average** 2X in the pectorals.

    – **Above average** 2X in the anterior deltoids.

    – **Above average** 2X in the triceps.

Above average NA/CNS potential.

In the above examples, at least two factors are above average and the others at least average. This would allow for more favorable results. It's difficult to determine which combinations would be more advantageous than others (i.e., above average NA/CNS + average skeletal leverage vs.

average NA/CNS potential + above average 2X in the pectorals and anterior deltoids). Regardless, the more above average one is, the greater their potential. On that, by comparison subject 4 who possesses five above average characteristics would be stronger than subject 3, who only possesses two above average characteristics.

FOUR FAVORABLE COMBINATIONS FOR DEMONSTRATING BELOW AVERAGE STRENGTH:

Conversely, the following four examples of average and/or below average would offer less favorable characteristics with which to perform a respectable 1-RM. Note that subject 7 possesses four below average characteristics. As a result, they would most likely be labeled the genetic trash bag of the four:

Subject 5: 1-RM = 255 pounds/116 kilograms.

Average muscle volume.

Below average skeletal leverage.

MU/fiber type quantity and distribution:

> – Average type 2X in the pectorals.

> – **Below average** 2X in the deltoids.

> – Average 2X in the triceps.

Average NA/CNS potential.

Subject 6: 1-RM =250 pounds/114 kilograms.

Average muscle volume.

Average skeletal leverage.

MU/fiber type quantity and distribution:

> – Average 2X in the pectorals.

> – **Below average** 2X in the anterior deltoids.

> – Average 2X in the triceps.

Below average NA/CNS potential.

Subject 7: 1-RM = 185 pounds/84 kilograms.

Below average muscle volume.

Below average skeletal leverage.

MU/fiber type quantity and distribution:

  – **Below average** 2X in the pectorals.

  – Average 2X in the deltoids.

  – Average 2X in the triceps.

Below average NA/CNS potential.

Subject 8: 1-RM =275 pounds/125 kilograms.

Average muscle volume.

Below Average skeletal leverage.

MU/fiber type quantity and distribution:

  – Average 2X in the pectorals.

  – Average 2X in the anterior deltoids.

  – Average 2X in the triceps.

Average NA/CNS potential.

Due to the many possible combinations it is difficult to single out one specific quality that accounts for one's exceptional (or deficient) ability to lift a relatively heavy 1-RM. Is it important to know exactly what accounts for the result? Not necessarily because the bottom line is for whatever reason(s), a person can either lift an average, above average, or below average amount of resistance in a 1-RM. However, when it comes to multiple rep sets in the forthcoming dissections of the 10-RM and 35-RM events, more factors are involved, particularly one's NA/CNS potential and MU/fiber quantity and distribution.

Pre-discussion Thoughts and Speculation on the 10-rm and 35-rm Sets to mmf

The performance and result of a 1-RM is the relatively simple to explain. When it comes to explaining multiple rep sets such as a 10-RM and 35-RM, more factors are involved which creates more diversity in possible outcomes. This is due in part to the aforementioned NA/CNS potential combined with MU/fiber type quantity and distribution among the working muscle groups. An additional factor to consider is rep performance regarding the movement velocity and cadence used to complete the prescribed number of reps. Those three factors together can significantly impact the amount of resistances used and the number of reps completed in those events.

REP VELOCITY AND CADENCE

Regarding rep velocity and cadence (time and manner of rep completion), the initial reps can be performed relatively faster due to less fatigue but the final reps slower due to more fatigue. Conversely, one can purposely move a submaximal resistance relatively slow in the initial fatigue-free reps, especially if the resistance is relatively light. This is where time under tension is a factor and not solely the number of reps performed. One could purposely move a lighter resistance as fast as possible (decreasing muscle tension = involving more momentum and increasing the risk of injury) and complete 20 reps in :35 (average of :01.75 per rep). They could also purposely move that same resistance slower (increasing muscle tension = involving less momentum and decreasing the risk of injury) and complete only 12 reps in :35 (average of :02.9 per rep).

Which approach is best? Both essentially recruit and fatigue a similar quantity of MUs/fibers, but the latter does not expose the muscle, tendon, and ligament structures to unnecessary stress and potential injury. Remember the force-velocity curve, Henneman's Principle, and energy systems involvement:

1. Greater force is generated at slower velocity. Therfore, improving strength with naturally slower velocity = increased force potential = enhanced power output (power = force x distance/time) in a safer manner..

> **NOTE:** Relative to imporving power for athletic performance, it is all about getting stronger in the weight room using safe and sensible protocols and practicing athletic skills as they will be required in competition at full "game" speed using sport-specific situations and contingencies unabated by resistance. The addition of resistance – even in modest amounts – violates the importance of exactness in the puruit of skill acquisition. Remember, specificity requires exactness, not almost or close to.

2. Regardless of velocity, MUs/fibers are recruited in order as the demand for force (greater effort) increases…type 1 ➡ type 2A ➡ type 2X. Therefore, there is no need to move resistances fast and increase injury risk. And it stands to reason the only way to move a resistance at a high velocity is if it is extremely light in the first place relative to one's maximum strength. And due to excess momentum relative to the force-velocity curve, moving too fast is a poor means of recruiting and fatiguing a significant quantity of MUs/fibers.

3. The rep velocity and cadence and total time under tension dictate where ATP comes from. Most resistance training involves primarily immediate stores, its replenishment via CK reaction, and glycolysis as effort extends past :15. The short term high effort, high MU/fiber recruitment events (under :12) tax immediate ATP stores and its quick replenishment via the CK reaction. The longer term moderately high effort, moderately high MU/fiber events (:12 to 1:00+) rely more upon the carbohydrate-dependent glycolytic system to generate ATP to complete them. So, even though it is standard practice to count reps as a means of documenting progression, always remember the bottom line is time under tension and intensity.

NA/CNS POTENTIAL

Regarding NA/CNS potential in conjunction with MU/fiber type quantity and distribution among the working muscle groups, many possibilities exist when performing multiple rep sets.

It's known a 1-RM is a slow-by-nature (ultra-heavy resistance!), all-out, maximum force generation event that is largely dictated by all genetic factors and skill.

If one has above average skeletal leverage, an above average quantity of type 2X MUs/fibers in the working muscle groups, and an above average ability to recruit many units of force in one instance they'll out-perform anyone lacking those exceptional genetics, period.

Possessing an above average NA/CNS potential means one can recruit a greater quantity of all MUs/fibers combined in one effort, hence a greater relative strength ability. However, because of that ability the reserve pool is diminished quicker during multiple rep sets against submaximal resistance. This is based on the fact that they are using relatively greater resistance in the multiple rep set as compared to one with an average or below average NA/CNS potential, thus more MUs/fibers will be recruited early and prone to more fatigue.

In example, a stronger person with an above average NA/CNS potential might use 300 lbs./136 kgs. (75% of a 400 lbs./182 kgs. 1-RM) and recruit and fatigue more MUs/fibers compared to a weaker person with a below average NA/CNS potential using only 244 lbs./111 kgs. (75% of a 325 lbs./148 kgs. 1-RM). The involvement of more MUs/fibers each rep leaves fewer units of force in the reserve pool. Using the same percentage of the 1-RM, fewer reps are consequently performed by the stronger person as compared to the weaker and below average NA/CNS person.

Multiple rep sets should also be performed to MMF safely with a controlled movement velocity and cadence, but their varied outcomes are contingent mostly on NA/CNS potential and MU/fiber type quantity and distribution in the working muscles. The amount of resistance used in them is dictated by those factors only. The exact percentage of their 1-RM that it equals is insignificant. The only important factor is the goal of achieving MMF, independent of whatever percentage of the 1-RM is used.

That pokes a lot of holes in programs that categorize reps into specific types of developments such as strength-only, power-only, strength-endurance, power-endurance, starting strength, explosive strength, etc. To say one to four reps only develop pure strength, eight to 12 reps are optimal to stimulate muscle growth, or lighter resistances in the 15 to 20 rep range moved "fast" to maximize power, is erroneous. Assuming that was proven as fact, what would performing six reps develop? What about 10 to 14 reps moved consciously slower and controlled? If a rep scheme that used 16 to 20 reps to MMF over a 10-week progressive plan resulted in visible muscle growth, what would that say for the recommended eight to 12 reps supposedly optimal for that goal?

Those commonly used terms like explosive power or pure strength are acceptable when describing one's visible force output during muscle contracting events, such as a power clean or a 1-RM bench press. However, it is not true to suggest those qualities can only be improved by solely using a specific set/rep scheme applicable to everyone. Whatever one's training status is during any force output event, it's dependent on their NA/CNS potential, MU/fiber type quantity and distribution, skill, and their conscious effort exuded. If a person with a 1-RM of 200 lbs./91 kgs. makes a conscious effort to move any amount of resistance as fast as possible, it will move as fast as their NA/CNS potential and MU/fiber type quantity and distribution allow. If they make a conscious effort to exert all-out, maximum force just to move a heavy resistance (i.e., 93% of their 1-RM), again the force output amount and velocity are also contingent on those factors.

In summary, one's ability to express force output - ranging from maximum and naturally slow to sub-maximum and potentially fast - is dependent on their genetic make-up and the conscious effort to exert. If they follow a progressive resistance training program that improves muscle force output within their genetic potential, those force expressions will be enhanced. Hence, there are no specific number of reps, range of reps, or percentages of a 1-RM that are optimal for the entire population. Each person is different genetically thus the optimal number of reps to perform for whatever goal they seek is contingent on what they possess. This is yet another point to understand regarding the "What's going on in there" as it highly suggests individualizing training plans that allow for more objective and attainable results.

THE ANATOMY OF A 10-RM

EXERCISE EXAMPLE: LEG PRESS FOR 10 REPS TO MOMENTARY MUSCLE FATIGUE.

ALL OTHER FACTORS BEING EQUAL...

MUSCLE FIBERS AND MOTOR UNITS

All three types of MUs/fibers – types 1, 2A, and 2X – will be involved in the 10-rep leg press event, but their recruitment will vary from the start to finish. Because the resistance used in the 10-RM is not maximal, not all will be recruited initially. The prime movers are the gluteal and quadriceps muscles (the hamstrings, calves, and hip adductors are also involved but this will focus on the prime movers).

Regarding body type, a greater volume of muscle in the acting muscles will increase the potential to use a heavier resistance for the 10-RM event due to a greater quantity of contractile tissue (i.e., stronger = higher 1-RM = a relatively heavier resistance used as compared to weaker person).

This is where the type and quantity of MUs/fibers have an impact. In the involved gluteals and quadriceps, possessing an above average quantity of type 2A MU's/fibers in at least one of them – and the other being average – it would be more advantageous as compared to a person possessing only average and/or below average in some combination.

THE NERVOUS SYSTEM

Through Henneman's Principle the recruitment of the necessary MUs/muscle fibers within one's NA/CNS potential from type 1 through the larger and stronger type 2X will receive CNS input. A significant quantity of type 2A and fewer 2X will be recruited initially due to the sub-maximal resistance, but as fatigue accumulates in both 2A and 2X MUs/fibers more units of force will be needed to complete the event.

The rate coding (firing rate) will also follow the pattern of recruitment through the type 1 ➡ type 2A ➡ type 2X order. Type 1 will initially be firing rapidly due to their immediate recruitment and then both the type 2A and 2X as they are critical to complete the event.

Because it is a sub-maximum resistance — yet still relatively heavy — the resistance movement velocity can potentially be faster than a 1-RM in the initial reps relative to the force-velocity curve. As fatigue begins to set in during the last three or so reps the velocity will naturally slow, especially at the weakest point of the exercise range of motion.

Compared to the 1-RM, a smaller reserve of MUs/fibers and resultant units of force will remain at the completion of the event. All type 1 will be available because none will be completely fatigued due to their greater endurance capacity. Remember, they are less force-producing but still assist in the reps as per Henneman's Principle. The type 2A reserve will be significantly depleted (approximately 75 to 80% fatigued) and the 2X pool will drop gradually to approximately 65 to 70% at the point of MMF. The remaining MU/fiber and U. O. F. reserve pool will be insufficient to perform an 11th rep.

CHEMICAL INTERACTIONS AT THE MOLECULAR LEVEL

The presence of minerals calcium, magnesium, potassium, and sodium, and the energy molecule ATP (all originating from dietary intake) will facilitate the actin and myosin cross bridging and maximize muscle contraction during the 10-RM effort.

ENERGY SYSTEMS FUELING MUSCLE

The 10-RM is an event that takes approximately :25 to :30+ to complete depending on rep velocity and cadence, any time spent resting in the lock-out position, and the distance the resistance must move through the exercise range of motion. It will rely upon stored ATP (:03), ATP resynthesized via the CK reaction (:12), and glycolysis (:12+) so the previous discussion on molecular level chemical interactions applies here.

CAUSES OF FATIGUE

The longer but intense process of completing the 10 reps will involve more MUs/fibers, thus more ATP coming from sources beyond only the immediate stores. The approximate :25 to :30 effort does tap into glycolysis, and fatigue will result from impairment of mechanisms of the excitation/coupling and cross-bridging processes in those highly recruited 2A and 2X MUs/fibers due to the peripheral fatigue factors, namely decreased ATP availability and metabolite accumulation (i.e.,

Ca+ overload, acidity). The more-enduring type 1 MUs/fibers might experience some impairment in excitation/coupling but will not become completely fatigued.

Central fatigue again will not be a concern in this one set of 10 reps. However, performing multiple sets (4+) of 10 reps with minimal rest between – a la circuit-type training – is likely to cause more central fatigue recovery concerns.

OTHER GENETIC FACTORS

Regarding skeletal leverage and NA/CNS potential, here is the essence of each from the *positive* viewpoint:

Shorter legs (levers) will offer a mechanical advantage to lift relatively heavier resistances in the 10-RM leg press. More favorable muscle insertions on bones will also make it a mechanical advantage to lift relatively heavier resistances.

NA/CNS potential is interesting when it comes to multiple rep sets. Much of the performance potential is contingent on 1) the quantity of each MU/fiber type in the acting muscles and 2) how many can be recruited each rep…either average, below average, or above average. For the ability to use a relatively heavy amount of resistance in a 10-RM leg press, two advantageous combinations would be:

1. Possessing an average NA/CNS potential and an above average quantity of type 2A MUs/fibers combined in gluteals and quadriceps. This would result in a slight above average 1-RM, but the due to the stronger and more enduring type 2A MUs/fibers, one could use a slightly heavier resistance in the event.

2. Possessing a below average NA/CNS potential and an average quantity of all MU/fiber types. This would result in a lesser 1-RM, but the ability to use a relatively heavier amount of resistance in the completion of the 10 reps.

TRAINING STATUS AND NUTRITION

Regarding training, a person who has never resistance trained or has not performed it in a while (i.e., detrained) will improve their 10-RM leg press relative to their genetic potential provided they follow a relevant progressive regimen. Also, if they are genetically gifted they would be able to demonstrate greater ability in the 10-RM (trained or untrained) compared to a less genetically endowed person (trained or untrained).

In any case, following a progressive resistance training regimen will improve the ability to perform more than 10 reps on the same leg press device with their initial 10-RM resistance due to an increased level of strength because being stronger allows for an improved display of local muscle endurance.

Some possible examples of improved local muscle endurance following a 60-day training period:

	10-RM (pounds/kilograms)	
	DAY 1	DAY 60
Non-trained/below average genetics	240/109	290/132
Non-trained/average genetics	310/141	360/164
Trained/average genetics	340/155	390/177
Trained/above average genetics	490/223	540/245

As for nutrition, consuming a standard diet should supply the minerals and ATP substrate among the associated leg pressing muscle groups needed for the performance of a 10-RM. If one has also consumed an adequate amount of protein over the course of their progressive training period, it will facilitate muscle growth and repair which will also increase the potential to use a heavier resistance for the 10-RM.

SKILL ACQUISITION AND ENHANCEMENT

Depending on the device used to perform the 10-RM leg press (plate-load or selectorized machine), the practice of using the same device in training will improve one's ability on that device. Comparing the amount of resistance used for a 10-RM on different leg press device is not as accurate due to design and leverage differences between each. Therefore, on that specific device, one will learn how to maximally recruit as many MUs/fibers possible within their NA/CNS potential to complete the 10 reps to MMF.

MOTIVATION AND MENTAL TOUGHNESS

Near the end of the set of 10 reps to MMF will be a challenge. One who is tolerant of temporary muscle discomfort and focused on achieving the 10-rep goal will be better prepared to complete it.

10-RM SUBJECT COMPARISONS

A more in-depth look at 10-RM leg press potential can be made by dissecting and comparing MU/fiber type quantity and NA/CNS potential of different subjects. Below is a breakdown of the characteristics and hypothetical 10-RM outcomes between eight subjects. Among the eight subjects some characteristics are the same while some are varied. Diagram 1 delineates all factors – CNS potential, the type and quantity of MUs in the involved muscles (MUs only, not U. O. .F.), the estimated 10-RM endurance (END.) and 1-RM strength (STR.) potentials, and the estimated amount of resistances that would be used for each. A detailed discussion of the eight subjects follows.

LEG PRESS 10-RM COMPARISON		MU TYPE, QUANTITY, AND DISTRIBUTION						END. POTENTIAL		STR. POTENTIAL		RESISTANCE		
		GLUTEALS			QUADRICEPS			1 + 2A		2A + 2X			% of 1-RM used	
SUBJECT	CNS POTENTIAL	TYPE 1	TYPE 2A	TYPE 2X	TYPE 1	TYPE 2A	TYPE 2X	GLUTES	QUADS	GLUTES	QUADS	10-RM		1-RM
1	Average 70%	Ave. 400	Ave. 280	Ave. 120	Ave. 500	Ave. 350	Ave. 150	680	850	400	500	280 lbs. 127 kgs.	80%	350 lbs. 159 kgs.
2	Average 70%	Ave. 400	Above Ave. 320	Below Ave. 80	Below Ave. 450	Ave. 350	Above Ave. 200	720	800	400	550	293 lbs. 133 kgs.	77.5%	378 lbs. 172 kgs.
3	Average 70%	Ave. 400	Ave. 280	Ave. 120	Above Ave. 550	Ave. 350	Below Ave. 100	680	900	400	450	266 lbs. 121 kgs.	82.5%	322 lbs. 146 kgs.
A	Above Average 74%	Ave. 400	Ave. 280	Ave. 120	Ave. 500	Ave. 350	Ave. 150	680	850	400	500	325 lbs. 148 kgs.	70%	464 lbs. 211 kgs.
B	Below Average 66%	Ave. 400	Ave. 280	Ave. 120	Below Ave. 450	Ave. 350	Above Ave. 200	680	800	400	550	242 lbs. 110 kgs.	87.5%	276 lbs. 125 kgs.
C	Above Average 74%	Above Ave. 440	Ave. 280	Below Ave. 80	Ave. 500	Above Ave. 400	Below Ave. 100	720	900	360	500	313 lbs. 142 kgs.	72.5%	432 lbs. 196 kgs.

Diagram 1: 10-RM comparisons

CONSTANTS

- Muscle volume and skeletal leverage are average for all subjects.
- Gluteals contain 800 total MUs (combined quantity of all type 1, 2A, and 2X).
- Quadriceps contain 1,000 total MUs.

VARIABLES

- NA/CNS potential.
- MU type and quantity distribution.
- Endurance potential.
- Strength potential.
- 1-RM resistance.
- Percentage of 1-RM used for 10-RM.
- 10-RM resistance.

Subject 1: overall average strength and endurance potential:

Average CNS/NA potential (70%).

MU type quantity and distribution:

– Gluteals - average of all types: 1 @ 400, 2A @ 280, and 2X @ 120.

– Quadriceps - average of all types: 1 @ 500, 2A @ 350, and 2X @ 150.

Strength potential (combined quantity of type 2A and 2X MUs):

– Gluteals @ 400.

– Quadriceps @ 500.

Endurance potential (combined quantity of type 1 and 2A MUs):

– Gluteals @ 680.

– Quadriceps @ 850.

1-RM leg press of 350 pounds/159 kilograms.

10-RM resistance used (80% of the 1-RM) – 280 pounds/127 kilograms.

Subject 2: overall slight above average strength and slight below average endurance potential:

Average CNS/NA potential (70%).

MU/fiber type quantity and distribution:

– Gluteals - average type 1 @ 400, **above average 2A @ 320,** and **below average 2X @ 80.**

– Quadriceps – **below average type 1 @ 450,** average 2A @ 350, and **above average 2X @ 200.**

Strength potential (combined quantity of type 2A and 2X MUs):

– Gluteals @ 400.

– Quadriceps @ **550.**

Endurance potential (combined quantity of type 1 and 2A MUs):

– Gluteals @ **720.**

– Quadriceps @ **800.**

1-RM leg press of 378 pounds/172 kilograms.

10-RM resistance used (77.5% of the 1-RM) – 293 pounds/133 kilograms.

Subject 3: overall slight below average strength and slight above average endurance potential:

Average CNS/NA potential (70%).

MU/fiber type quantity and distribution:

- Gluteals - average of all types: 1 @ 400, 2A @ 280, and 2X @ 120.
- Quadriceps – **above average type 1 @ 550**, average 2A @ 350, and **below average 2X @ 100**.

Strength potential (combined quantity of type 2A and 2X MUs):

- Gluteals @ 400.
- Quadriceps @ **450**.

Endurance potential (combined quantity of type 1 and 2A MUs):

- Gluteals @ 680.
- Quadriceps @ **900**.

1-RM leg press of 322 pounds/146 kilograms.

10-RM resistance used (82.5% of the 1-RM) – 266 pounds/121 kilograms.

Subject A: overall above average strength and below average endurance potential.

Above Average CNS/NA potential (74%).

MU/fiber type quantity and distribution:

- Gluteals – average of all types: 1 @ 400, 2A @ 280, and 2X @ 120.
- Quadriceps - average of all types: 1 @ 500, 2A @ 350, and 2X @ 150.

Strength potential (combined quantity of type 2A and 2X MUs):

- Gluteals @ 400.

- Quadriceps @ 500.

Endurance potential (combined quantity of type 1 and 2A MUs):

- Gluteals @ 680.

- Quadriceps @ 850.

1-RM leg press of 464 pounds/211 kilograms.

10-RM resistance used (70% of the 1-RM) – 325 pounds/148 kilograms.

Subject B: overall slight below above average strength (due to the below average NA/CNS potential) and slight above average endurance potential

Below Average CNS/NA potential (66%).

MU/fiber type quantity and distribution:

- Gluteals – average of all types: 1 @ 400, 2A @ 280, and 2X @ 120.

- Quadriceps – **below average type 1 @ 450**, average 2A @ 350, and **above average 2X @ 200**.

Strength potential (combined quantity of type 2A and 2X MUs):

- Gluteals @ 400.

- Quadriceps @ **550**.

Endurance potential (combined quantity of type 1 and 2A MUs):

- Gluteals @ 680.

- Quadriceps @ **800**.

1-RM leg press of 276 pounds/125 kilograms.

10-RM resistance used (87.5% of the 1-RM) – 242 pounds/110 kilograms.

Subject C: overall slight above average strength (below average of type 2X in both muscles *do not* offset the above average NA/CNS potential) and slight below average endurance potential

Above Average CNS/NA potential (74%).

MU/fiber type quantity and distribution:

- Gluteals – **above average type 1 @ 440**, average 2A @ 280, and **below average 2X @ 80.**

- Quadriceps – average type 1 @ 500, **above average 2A @ 400**, and **below average 2X @ 100.**

Strength potential (combined quantity of type 2A and 2X MUs):

- Gluteals @ **360.**

- Quadriceps @ 500.

Endurance potential (combined quantity of type 1 and 2A MUs):

- Gluteals @ **720.**

- Quadriceps @ **900.**

1-RM leg press of 432 pounds/196 kilograms.

10-RM resistance used (72.5% of the 1-RM) – 313 pounds/142 kilograms.

DISCUSSION

Subject 1 has an average NA/CNS potential, an average quantity of all MUs/fibers, thus can recruit an average quantity of all MUs/fibers each rep. Their ability is then average strength, endurance, and an average MU/fiber reserve. They can perform the 10-RM with 80% of the 1-RM.

Subject 2 has an average NA/CNS potential, an **above average** quantity of important type 2A and 2X MUs/fibers *combined* in the gluteals and quadriceps (**above-below**-average-**above**), thus they can recruit a **slight above average** total quantity of 2A and 2X each rep which equals a **slight above average strength**. A **slight below average endurance** reserve is available due to the balance between the **above average** 2A in the gluteals and **below average** type 1 in the quadriceps. They must use a lighter resistance to perform a 10-RM with 77.5% of 1-RM due to their **slight above average strength** as compared to subject 1.

Subject 3 has an average NA/CNS potential, an average quantity of all MUs/fibers in the gluteals, but a **below average** quantity of 2A and 2X MUs/fibers *combined* in the quadriceps (average-**below average**), thus can recruit a **slight below average** quantity of 2A and 2X each rep which equals a **slight below average strength** but a **slight above average endurance** reserve due to and **above average** quantity of type 1 MUs/fibers in the quadriceps. They will have a lower 1-RM but will be able to use a slightly heavier resistance (82.5%) for the 10-RM event compared to subject 1.

Subject A has an **above average NA/CNS potential** (big advantage for demonstrating strength) and an average quantity of all MUs/fibers combined, thus they can recruit an **above average** quantity of all MUs/fibers each rep. That equals **above average strength** and **below average endurance** potential. Due to their above average strength (and thus fewer total MUs/fibers in reserve), they can only perform the 10-RM with 70% of the 1-RM.

Subject B has a **below average NA/CNS potential** (big advantage for endurance) and an average quantity of all MUs/fibers combined in the gluteals and quadriceps (quadriceps @ **below**-average-**above**), thus they can only recruit a **below average** quantity of total MUs/fibers. That equals a **slight below average strength** but a **slight above average endurance** potential. With the below average ability to recruit MUs/fibers – but an **above average** quantity of 2X in the quadriceps – they would have a much lower 1-RM compared to subject B but could use a greater amount of resistance for the 10-RM (87.5% vs. 70%).

Subject C possesses an **above average NA/CNS potential**, a *combined* **above average** type 1 and 2A in the gluteals and quadriceps (**above**-average-average-**above**), and a *combined* below average of 2A and 2X (average-**below-above-below**). Their strength potential would probably be **slight above average** (better NA/CNS potential + very low overall 2X) like subject B, but their endurance potential would be **slight below average** due to the more enduring type 1 and 2A MUs/fibers. Therefore, the amount of resistance used in the 10RM would be closer to subject A (72.5% vs. 70%) due to their lower 1-RM.

THE ANATOMY OF A 35-RM

EXERCISE EXAMPLE: PLATE-LOAD ROW (HORIZONTAL ROW).

ALL OTHER FACTORS BEING EQUAL...

MUSCLE FIBERS AND MOTOR UNITS

Because performing 35 reps to muscle fatigue requires a relatively lighter resistance than the 10-RM, from the initial reps to approximately 25 will be driven solely by type 1 and 2A MUs/fibers in the primary activated muscles - the latissimus dorsi "lats" and biceps brachii (the trapezius, rhomboids, external rotator cuff muscles, posterior deltoids, and two other elbow flexors, the brachioradialis and brachialis are also involved but this will focus on the prime movers). The low tension created by that amount will not activate the high threshold 2X MUs/fibers until they are needed deep into the set when fatigue begins to take a toll.

Regarding body type, a greater volume of muscle in those muscles will increase the potential to use a heavier resistance for the 35-RM event due to a greater quantity of contractile tissue. Remember, more strength potential = greater local muscle endurance potential = a relatively heavier resistance used as compared to weaker person, all other factors being equal.

Again, the type and quantity of MUs/fibers factor into the amount of muscle volume. In the involved lats and biceps, possessing an above average quantity of 2A MUs/fibers in at least one of them – and neither being below average – would be more advantageous as compared to a person possessing only an average and/or below average quantity in some combination.

THE NERVOUS SYSTEM

Through Henneman's Principle and one's NA/CNS potential, the recruitment of the necessary MUs/fibers and resultant units of force from type 1 to type 2A, then the 2X near the end, receive CNS input. Remember, high threshold 2X MUs/fibers are only activated in large tension-creating situations and the amount of resistance required for this lengthy event precludes them from being recruited early on.

The rate coding (firing rate) will also follow the pattern of recruitment through the type 1 ➡ type 2A ➡ type 2X order. Type 1 will initially be firing rapidly due to their earlier recruitment and then type 2A and 2X as more are needed in the latter reps to keep the resistance moving as fatigue increases.

Because of this lighter sub-maximum resistance - but approximately at least 50% of the 1-RM for most people...still relatively heavy - the resistance movement velocity can be faster initially compared to the 10-RM event relative to the force-velocity curve. As fatigue begins to set in during the last five or so reps, the velocity will naturally slow even more, especially at the weakest point of the exercise range of motion.

In this extended set an even smaller reserve of total MUs/fibers and U. O. F. will remain at its completion. Because the longer-in-time 35-RM (1:30+) crosses into the aerobic energy system zone, glycolysis will be producing most of the ATP needed for continual force output, thus the intermediate 2A MUs/fibers will be completely depleted. The need to continue force output will finally tap into the 2X pool in the latter and now more tension-producing reps. In the end the reserve pool of 2X will be approximately 40 to 45% still available. Peripheral fatigue will be more prevalent due to the greater accumulation of lactic acid and other metabolites from the more relied upon glycolytic system. Hence, a 36th rep cannot be completed.

CHEMICAL INTERACTIONS AT THE MOLECULAR LEVEL

The presence of minerals calcium, magnesium, potassium, and sodium, and the energy molecule ATP (all originating from dietary intake) will facilitate the actin and myosin cross bridging and maximize muscle contraction during the 35-RM effort.

ENERGY SYSTEMS FUELING MUSCLE

The 35-RM is an event that takes approximately 1:30 to 1:45+ to complete, depending on rep velocity and cadence, any time spent resting in the lock-out position, and the distance the resistance must move through the exercise range of motion. It will rely upon stored ATP (:03), ATP resynthesized via the CK reaction (:12), then heavily on glycolysis (:12+), especially around the 1:00 point. The high dependence on the type 2A intermediate MUs/fibers past that point will begin obtaining more ATP from the aerobic system as it becomes more available to assist up through the 35th and final rep.

CAUSES OF FATIGUE

The much longer but still intense process of completing the 35 reps will involve more repetitive use of all the MUs/fibers recruited, thus more ATP coming from the now-important glycolytic system. The approximate 1:30 to 1:45 effort creates more peripheral fatigue resulting in impairment of mechanisms from the excitation/coupling process to cross-bridging due to muscle acidity, a decrease in available ATP at required sites, and a disruption of calcium movement mainly in the type 2A MUs/fibers and some 2X. The more-enduring type 1 MUs/fibers will experience more impairment in excitation/coupling but will not become completely fatigued.

Central fatigue may be a minor concern in this one set of 35 reps. However, performing multiple 35-RM sets will possibly elicit some central fatigue if one is performing two or three sets, even with adequate recovery time between them. Performing many multiple sets (3+) of 35 reps with minimal rest between – a la circuit-type training – is will cause a greater central fatigue recovery concern.

OTHER GENETIC FACTORS

Regarding skeletal leverage and NA/CNS potential, here is the essence of each from the *positive* viewpoint:

Shorter arms (levers) will offer a mechanical advantage to lift relatively heavier resistances in the 35-RM plate-load row. More favorable muscle insertions on bones will also offer a mechanical advantage to lift relatively heavier resistances during the 35 reps.

NA/CNS potential in an extended set of 35 reps to MMF can also vary. Like any multiple rep set, one's performance potential is contingent on 1) the quantity of each MU/fiber type in the acting muscles and 2) how many can be recruited each rep…either average, below average, or above average.

For the ability to use a relatively heavy amount of resistance in a 35-RM plate-load row, two advantageous combinations would be:

1. Possessing an average NA/CNS potential, an above average quantity of type 2A MUs/fibers combined in the lats and bi-

ceps, with neither of those muscles being below average. This would result in a slightly above average 1-RM, but due to the both strong/enduring type 2A and the fact type 1 also contribute, one could use a slightly heavier resistance in the event.

2. Possessing a below average NA/CNS potential and an average quantity of all MU/fiber types, or a slight above average quantity of both type 2A and type 1 combined. This would result in a lesser 1-RM, but the ability to use a relatively heavier amount of resistance.

TRAINING STATUS AND NUTRITION

Regarding training, a person who has never resistance trained or has not performed it in a while (i.e., detrained) will improve their 35-RM plate load row relative to their genetic potential provided they follow a relevant progressive regimen. Also, if they are genetically gifted they would be able to demonstrate greater ability in the 35-RM (trained or untrained) compared to a less genetically endowed person (trained or untrained). In any case, following a progressive resistance training regimen will improve the ability to perform more than 35 reps on the same plate-load row device with their initial 35-RM resistance because of the improved strength. Being stronger allows for an improved display of local muscle endurance.

Some possible examples of improved local muscle endurance following a 60-day training period:

	35-RM (pounds/kilograms)	
	DAY 1	DAY 60
Non-trained/below average genetics	135/61	160/73
Non-trained/average genetics	160/73	190/86
Trained/average genetics	185/84	215/98
Trained/above average genetics	240/109	275/125

As for nutrition, consuming a standard diet should supply the minerals and ATP substrate needed for the performance of a 35-RM among the associated upper body pulling muscle groups. If one has also consumed an adequate amount of protein over the course of their progressive training period, it will facilitate muscle growth and repair which will also increase the potential to use a heavier resistance for the 35-RM.

SKILL ACQUISITION AND ENHANCEMENT

Depending on the device used to perform the 35-RM plate-load row (in this case, a plate-load machine but one could use a selectorized machine, dumbbells or a barbell), the practice of using the same device in training will optimize one's potential to complete it with the greatest amount of resistance possible. One will learn how to maximally recruit as many MUs/fibers possible within their NA/CNS potential to complete the 35 reps to muscle fatigue.

MOTIVATION AND MENTAL TOUGHNESS

Performing 35 reps is a grind. As muscle fatigue accumulates – especially in the final five to seven reps – one must remain focused on the task of achieving true momentary muscle fatigue. One who is tolerant of temporary muscle discomfort and able to stay focused will be better able to complete the task.

35-RM SUBJECT COMPARISONS

A more in-depth look at 35-RM plate-load row potential can be made by dissecting and comparing MU/fiber type quantity and NA/CNS potential of different subjects. Below is a breakdown of the characteristics and hypothetical 35-RM outcomes between eight subjects. Diagram 2 delineates all factors – CNS potential, the type and quantity of MUs in the involved muscles (MUs only, not U. O. F.), the estimated 35-RM (END.) and 1-RM (STR.) potentials, and the estimated amount of resistances used for each. A detailed discussion of each of the eight subjects follows.

PLATE-LOAD ROW 35-RM COMPARISON		MU TYPE, QUANTITY, AND DISTRIBUTION						END. POTENTIAL		STR. POTENTIAL		RESISTANCE		
		LATISSIMUS DORSI			BICEPS BRACHII			1 + 2A		2A + 2X				
SUBJECT	CNS POTENTIAL	TYPE 1	TYPE 2A	TYPE 2X	TYPE 1	TYPE 2A	TYPE 2X	LATS	BICEPS	LATS	BICEPS	35-RM	% of 1-RM used	1-RM
4	Average 70%	Ave. 600	Ave. 420	Ave. 180	Ave. 175	Ave. 122	Ave. 53	1,020	297	600	175	151 lbs. 69 kgs.	55%	275 lbs. 125 kgs.
5	Average 70%	Ave. 600	Above Ave. 480	Below Ave. 120	Ave. 175	Ave. 122	Ave. 53	1,080	297	600	175	147 lbs. 67 kgs.	58%	253 lbs. 115 kgs.
6	Average 70%	Ave. 600	Below Ave. 360	Above Ave. 240	Below Ave. 158	Ave. 122	Above Ave. 70	960	280	600	192	156 lbs. 71 kgs.	49%	319 lbs. 145 kgs.
D	Above Average 74%	Ave. 600	Ave. 420	Ave. 180	Ave. 175	Ave. 122	Ave. 53	1,020	297	600	175	167 lbs. 76 kgs.	46%	364 lbs. 166 kgs.
E	Below Average 66%	Below Ave. 540	Ave. 420	Above Ave. 240	Above Ave. 193	Ave. 122	Below Ave. 35	960	315	660	157	127 lbs. 58 kgs.	64%	198 lbs. 90 kgs.
F	Above Average 74%	Ave. 600	Ave. 420	Ave. 180	Ave. 175	Below Ave. 105	Above Ave. 70	1,020	280	600	175	167 lbs. 76 kgs.	43%	389 lbs. 177 kgs.

Diagram 2: 35-RM Comparison

CONSTANTS

- Muscle volume and skeletal leverage are average for all subjects.

- Latissimus Dorsi contain 1,200 total MU (combined quantity of all type 1, 2A, and 2X).

- Biceps brachii contain 350 total MUs.

VARIABLES

- NA/CNS potential.

- MU type quantity and distribution.

- Endurance potential.

- Strength potential.

- 1-RM resistance.

- Percentage of 1-RM used for 35-RM.

- 35-RM resistance.

Subject 4: overall average strength and endurance potential

Average CNS/NA potential (70%).

MU/fiber type quantity and distribution:

  – Latissimus Dorsi – average of all types: 1 @ 600, 2A @ 420, and 2X @ 180.

  – Biceps Brachii – average of all type: 1 @ 175, 2A @ 122 2A, 2X @ 53.

Strength potential (combined quantity of type 2A and 2X MUs):

  – Latissimus Dorsi @ 600.

  – Biceps Brachii @ 175.

Endurance potential (combined quantity of type 1 and 2A MUs):

  – Latissimus Dorsi @ 1,020.

  – Biceps Brachii @ 297.

1-RM Plate-load row of 275 pounds/125 kilograms.

35-RM resistance used (55% of the 1-RM) – 151 pounds/69 kilograms.

Subject 5: overall slight below average strength and slight above average endurance potential

Average CNS/NA potential (70%).

MU/fiber type quantity and distribution:

  – Latissimus Dorsi – average type 1 @ 600, **above average 2A @ 480**, and **below average 2X @ 120**.

  – Biceps brachii – average of all type: 1 @ 175, 2A @ 122 2A, 2X @ 53.

Strength potential (combined quantity of type 2A and 2X MUs):

  – Latissimus Dorsi @ 600.

  – Biceps Brachii @ 175.

Endurance potential (combined quantity of type 1 and 2A MUs):

  – Latissimus Dorsi @ **1,080**.

  – Biceps Brachii @ 297.

1-RM plate-load row of 253 pounds/115 kilograms.

10-RM resistance used (58% of the 1-RM) – 147 pounds/67 kilograms.

Subject 6: overall above average strength and below average endurance potential

Average CNS/NA potential (70%).

MU/fiber type quantity and distribution:

- – Latissimus Dorsi – average type 1 @ 600, **below average 2A @ 360**, and **above average 2X @ 240**.

- – Biceps brachii – **below average type 1 @ 158**, average 2A @ 122, and **above average 2X @ 70**.

Strength potential (combined quantity of type 2A and 2X MUs):

- – Latissimus Dorsi @ 600.

- – Biceps Brachii @ **192**.

Endurance potential (combined quantity of type 1 and 2A MUs):

- – Latissimus Dorsi @ **960**.

- – Biceps Brachii @ **280**.

1-RM plate-load row of 319 pounds/145 kilograms.

10-RM resistance used (49% of the 1-RM) – 156 pounds/71 kilograms.

Subject D: overall above average strength (due to 74% NA) and below average endurance potential

Above Average CNS/NA potential (74%).

MU/fiber type quantity and distribution:

- – Latissimus Dorsi – average of all types: 1 @ 600, 2A @ 420, and 2X @ 180.

- – Biceps brachii – average of all type: 1 @ 175, 2A @ 122 2A, 2X @ 53.

Strength potential (combined quantity of type 2A and 2X MUs):

- Latissimus Dorsi @ 600.
- Biceps Brachii @ 175.

Endurance potential (combined quantity of type 1 and 2A MUs):

- Latissimus Dorsi @ 1,020.
- Biceps Brachii @ 297.

1-RM Plate-load row of 364 pounds/166 kilograms.

35-RM resistance used (46% of the 1-RM) – 167 pounds/76 kilograms.

Subject E: overall below average strength (due to 66% NA) and above average endurance potential

Below average CNS/NA potential (66%).

MU/fiber type quantity and distribution:

- Latissimus Dorsi – **below average type 1 @ 540**, average 2A @ 420, and **above average 2X @ 240**.
- Biceps brachii – **above average type 1 @ 193**, average 2A @ 122 2A, and **below average 2X @ 35**.

Strength potential (combined quantity of type 2A and 2X MUs):

- Latissimus Dorsi @ **660**.
- Biceps Brachii @ **157**.

Endurance potential (combined quantity of type 1 and 2A MUs):

- Latissimus Dorsi @ **960**.
- Biceps Brachii @ **315**.

1-RM Plate-load row of 198 pounds/90 kilograms.

35-RM resistance used (64% of the 1-RM) – 127 pounds/58 kilograms.

Subject F: overall way above average strength (due to 74% NA) and way below average endurance potential

Above average CNS/NA potential (74%).

MU/fiber type quantity and distribution:

- – Latissimus Dorsi – average of all types: 1 @ 600, 2A @ 420, and 2X @ 180.
- – Biceps brachii – average of type @ 175, **below average 2A @ 105, and above average 2X @ 70.**

Strength potential (combined quantity of type 2A and 2X MUs):

- – Latissimus Dorsi @ 600.
- – Biceps Brachii @ 175.

Endurance potential (combined quantity of type 1 and 2A MUs):

- – Latissimus Dorsi @ 1,020.
- – Biceps Brachii @ **280.**

1-RM Plate-load row of 389 pounds/177 kilograms.

35-RM resistance used (43% of the 1-RM) – 167 pounds/76 kilograms.

DISCUSSION

Subject 4 has an average NA/CNS potential, an average quantity of all MUs/fibers, thus can recruit an average quantity of all MUs/fibers each rep = average endurance and strength, and average MU/fiber reserve. They can perform the 35-RM with 55% of the 1-RM.

Subject 5 has an average NA/CNS potential, but overall a **slight below average strength** and **slight above average endurance**. The only factors that create this potential is the *combined* 2A (**above average**) and 2X (**below average**) MUs/fibers in the Latissimus Dorsi (Lats) which would give the light edge to better endurance than strength as compared to subject 4. They could use a heavier amount of resistance for the 35-RM (58% 1-RM) as compared to subject 4.

Subject 6 has an average NA/CNS potential but a combination of MUs/fibers that makes them stronger but less enduring. Their **above average strength** is due to a combined above average 2A and 2X in the Lats (**below-above**) and Biceps Brachii (average-**above**). Their **below average endurance** would require a lighter 35-RM resistance of approximately 49% of a 1-RM.

Subject D has an **above average NA/CNS potential** and thus an **above average strength** and **below average endurance** potential. Their MU/ fiber type quantity and distribution is overall average thus their NA/

CNS potential dictates their ability. 46% (167 lbs./76 kgs.) of the 1-RM (364 lbs./166 kgs.) could be used for the 35-RM.

Subject E possesses a **below average NA/CNS potential**, hence **below average strength** and **above average endurance** potential. This holds true even when factoring in the combined MU/fiber quantity and distribution among the working muscles (endurance *combined* @ **below**-average-**above**-average and strength *combined* @ average-**above**-average-**below**). The below average NA/CNS potential trumps those combinations, thus 64% of the 1-RM can be used for the 35-RM event.

Subject F like subject D, has an **above average NA/CNS potential**. In this case – in addition to a combined above average 2A and 2X MUs/fibers (average-average-average-**above**) – they have a **way above average strength** potential, but consequently a **way below average endurance** potential (average-average-average-**below**). They will only be able to use 43% of the 1-RM to obtain a 35-RM.

Motor Unit Recruitment and Fatigue Simplified: Motor Units & Units of Force Combined

Assigning a unit of force (U. O. F.) value to each of the three MU/fiber types can better help understand their contribution relative to any resistance training situation. We know a low force activity (i.e., pressing a light weight overhead) requires fewer overall MUs/fibers and less force compared to a high force activity (i.e., pressing a heavy weight overhead). Therefore, each of the smaller MUs/fibers exert a lesser amount of force as compared to each of the larger ones. In this discussion the smaller and weaker type 1 MUs/fibers have been assigned a U. O. F. value of one. The intermediate type 2A have a value of two. The larger and stronger type 2X have a value of three. Therefore:

Type 1 = 1,000 MUs total and 1,000 total U. O. F. (1,000 x 1).

2A = 500 MUs total and 1,000 total U. O. F. (500 x 2).

2X = 500 MUs total and 1,500 total U. O. F. (500 x 3).

The diagram 3 on the following page depicts the hypothetical U. O. F. needed to complete a 10-RM. The quantity of MUs/fibers recruited during the 1st, 5th, and 10th rep are noted regarding 1) the U. O. F. being used to perform that rep and 2) the U. O. F. that have been recruited and fatigued before that rep.

- Total number of all MUs = 2,000. Total amount of U. O. F. = 3,500.

- 70% NA/CNS potential = 2,450 U. O. F. maximum (70% of 3,500).

- Total amount of U. O. F. needed to complete each rep of the 10-RM = approximately 1,950 (submaximal resistance, therefore not all 2,450 will be required each rep).

10-RM	KEY:	O = NOT RECRUITED, NOT FATIGUED	
		⊗ = RECRUITED, NOT FATIGUED	⊗ = RECRUITMENT LIMIT
		● = RECRUITED AND FATIGUED	

- Not recruited, not fatigued = not involved in the rep. Completely dormant.

- Recruited, not fatigued = used in the rep, but not fatigued (able to assist in further reps).

- Recruitment limit = the portion of those MUs/fibers recruited to meet the 1,950 total to complete the rep.

- Recruited and fatigued = those MUs/fibers that were recruited, fatigued, and now unable to assist in further reps.

MOTOR UNIT RECRUITMENT - UNITS OF FORCE (U. O. F.)

FROM TYPE 1, 2A, and 2X FIBERS

Total number of MUs = **2,000**   [Type 1 = 1,000 + 2A = 500 + 2X = 500]

UNITS OF FORCE:		70% NA/CNS Potential
TYPE 1 = 1	TYPE I = 1,000 U. O. F. (1,000 MUs x 1)	3,500 total U. O. F.
TYPE 2A = 2	TYPE 2A = 1,000 U. O. F. (500 MUs x 2)	1-RM = 2,450 U. O. F. (70% of 3,500)
TYPE 2X = 3	TYPE 2X = 1,500 U. O. F. (500 MUs x 3)	

The 10-RM requires at least 1,950 U. O. F. each rep (Approx. 80% of the 2,450 total)

10-RM

KEY:
- O = NOT RECRUITED, NOT FATIGUED
- ⊗ = RECRUITED, NOT FATIGUED   ⊗ = RECRUITMENT LIMIT
- ● = RECRUITED AND FATIGUED

REP #1

TYPE I FIBERS

⊗ ⊗	⊗ ⊗	⊗ ⊗	⊗ ⊗	⊗ ⊗	⊗ ⊗	⊗ ⊗	⊗ ⊗	⊗ ⊗	⊗ ⊗
MOTOR UNITS: 50 50	50 50	50 50	50 50	50 50	50 50	50 50	50 50	50 50	50 50
UNITS OF FORCE: 50 50	50 50	50 50	50 50	50 50	50 50	50 50	50 50	50 50	50 50
TOTAL U. O. F.: 100	200	300	400	500	600	700	800	900	1,000

TYPE 2A FIBERS

⊗ ⊗	⊗ ⊗	⊗ ⊗	⊗ O	O O
MOTOR UNITS: 50 50	50 50	50 50	50 50	50 50
UNITS OF FORCE: 100 100	100 100	100 100	100 100	100 100
TOTAL U. O. F.: 200	400	600	800	1,000

Units of force to meet the minimum 1,950 requirement:

TYPE 2X FIBERS

⊗ ⊗	O O	O O	O O	O O
MOTOR UNITS: 50 50	50 50	50 50	50 50	50 50
UNITS OF FORCE: 150 100	150 150	150 150	150 150	150 150
TOTAL U. O. F.: 300	600	900	1,200	1,500

1,000 x 1
700 x 2A
250 x 2X

REP #5

TYPE I FIBERS

⊗ ⊗	⊗ ⊗	⊗ ⊗	⊗ ⊗	⊗ ⊗	⊗ ⊗	⊗ ⊗	⊗ ⊗	⊗ ⊗	⊗ ⊗
MOTOR UNITS: 50 50	50 50	50 50	50 50	50 50	50 50	50 50	50 50	50 50	50 50
UNITS OF FORCE: 50 50	50 50	50 50	50 50	50 50	50 50	50 50	50 50	50 50	50 50
TOTAL U. O. F.: 100	200	300	400	500	600	700	800	900	1,000

TYPE 2A FIBERS

● ●	● ●	⊗ ⊗	⊗ ⊗	⊗ ⊗
MOTOR UNITS: 50 50	50 50	50 50	50 50	50 50
UNITS OF FORCE: 100 100	100 100	100 100	100 100	100 100
TOTAL U. O. F.: 200	400	600	800	1,000

Units of force to meet the minimum 1,950 requirement:

TYPE 2X FIBERS

● ●	● ⊗	⊗ ⊗	O O	O O
MOTOR UNITS: 50 50	50 50	50 50	50 50	50 50
UNITS OF FORCE: 150 150	150 150	150 50	150 150	150 150
TOTAL U. O. F.: 300	600	900	1,200	1,500

1,000 x 1
600 x 2A
350 x 2X

REP #10

TYPE I FIBERS

⊗ ⊗	⊗ ⊗	⊗ ⊗	⊗ ⊗	⊗ ⊗	⊗ ⊗	⊗ ⊗	⊗ ⊗	⊗ ⊗	⊗ ⊗
MOTOR UNITS: 50 50	50 50	50 50	50 50	50 50	50 50	50 50	50 50	50 50	50 50
UNITS OF FORCE: 50 50	50 50	50 50	50 50	50 50	50 50	50 50	50 50	50 50	50 50
TOTAL U. O. F.: 100	200	300	400	500	600	700	800	900	1,000

TYPE 2A FIBERS

● ●	● ●	● ●	⊗ ⊗	⊗ ⊗
MOTOR UNITS: 50 50	50 50	50 50	50 50	50 50
UNITS OF FORCE: 100 100	100 100	100 100	100 100	100 100
TOTAL U. O. F.: 200	400	600	800	1,000

Units of force to meet the minimum 1,950 requirement:

TYPE 2X FIBERS

● ●	● ●	● ⊗	⊗ ⊗	⊗ O
MOTOR UNITS: 50 50	50 50	50 50	50 50	50 50
UNITS OF FORCE: 150 150	150 150	150 150	150 150	100 150
TOTAL U. O. F.: 300	600	900	1,200	1,500

1,000 x 1
400 x 2A
550 x 2X

TOTAL MUs FATIGUED = 0/1,000 Type 1   300/500 2A   250/500 2X

Diagram 3: Simplified MU & U.O.F. Recruitment & Fatigue – 10-RM

Units Of Force Used: Start – Mid-point – End.

REP #1:

- All 1,000 U. O. F. of type 1 are used but not fatigued due to their higher endurance capacity. In line with Henneman's Principle they are the first MUs/fibers recruited due to the heavy nature of the event.

- The 10-RM is a relatively demanding event; thus 700 U. O. F. are contributed by the type 2A, but they are not fatigued. 300 U. O. F. are unrecruited.

- 250 U. O. F. are contributed by the 2X and are also not completely fatigued at the conclusion of the first rep. 1,250 U. O. F. remain available.

REP #5:

- Again, all 1,000 U. O. F. of the type 1 are used but remain unfatigued.

- 400 2A U. O. F. are unavailable (they're fatigued) to complete the 5th rep. The remaining 600 U. O. F. are recruited but remain unfatigued at this point.

- More type 2X U. O. F. are needed (350) as 450 have been fatigued. The 350 used are unfatigued and a reserve of 700 U. O. F. remain unrecruited.

REP #10:

- All 1,000 U. O. F. are still available from type 1 and again contribute. Remember, they are needed but have that higher endurance, so they do not completely fatigue.

- The diminished pool of 2A U. O. F. is down to 400 and all must be recruited to finish the job. 600 U. O. F. have been totally fatigued to this point.

- Naturally, the higher threshold type 2X are called upon due to the depleted 2A pool. At this point 750 type 2X U. O. F. are completely fatigued, 550 are needed to assist, and believe it or not, 200 U. O. F. remain untouched:

  - Total 2X U. O. F. = 1,500.

- 1,500 - 750 fatigued = 750 available.

- 750 available - 550 being used for the 10th rep = 200 in reserve.

At the conclusion of the 10th rep and the attempt for an 11th, there is a lack of overall "fresh" U. O. F. from all three MU/fiber types needed to complete that rep (1,950). Hence, the set is terminated.

MORE DETAILED MU RECRUITMENT-FATIGUE + ENERGY SYSTEMS

The following diagrams are hypothetical. They are intended to depict the recruitment and fatigue of MUs (not U.O.F.) in a 1-RM, 10-RM, and 35-RM regarding their initial tension, accumulating fatigue, the recruitment of more MUs in compliance with Henneman's Principle, rate coding, and energy system involvement to the point where peripheral fatigue (MMF) halts the process within a 70% NA/CNS potential and a MU quantity of 750 type 1, 488 type 2A, and 262 type 2X distributed in one muscle only.

The purpose of the finer details in the rep-by-rep sequence is to illustrate the convergence of neuromuscular system activity and energy system interaction from the first to last rep. They may not be completely accurate regarding the precise contribution of ATP supplied at each second/during each rep. However, it does provide a plausible overview of "what's going on in there" to better understand the underpinnings of resistance training sets performed to MMF.

The highlighted color-coded text below refers to color-coded sections on the following 1-RM, 10-RM, and 35-RM hypothetical recruitment-fatigue-energy systems diagrams. They address all components and factors effecting the set on a rep-by-rep basis and summarize set performance.

The motor unit recruitment – fatigue + energy systems interplay is based on the hypothetical average quantity of 1,500 total combined and an average neurological ability/CNS potential of 70% (in a maximum effort only 70% of each type can be recruited). The average quantity is broken down as 50% type 1, 33% type 2A, and 17% type 2X. It depicts one muscle group involved in the exercise as a means of simplification. If the exercise is a single joint (i.e., chest fly) it would apply to the pectorals only (even though the anterior deltoid is involved). Similarly, if the exercise is multiple joint (i.e., overhead press) it would apply to the deltoids (even though the trapezius and triceps are involved). Understand each of these muscles – along with other supporting secondary muscles – could have varied characteristics in terms of the quantity and distribution of the three MUs/fiber types, as well as different muscle volumes and skeletal factors (i.e., bone length and muscle insertion points).

The MU/fiber recruitment process would occur as follows as the demand of the event proceeds and increases from a lower to a higher effort:

Recruit type 1 ➡ recruit more type 1 ➡ higher rate coding of type 1 ➡ recruit type 2A ➡ recruit more type 2A ➡ higher rate coding of type 2A ➡ recruit type 2X ➡ recruit more 2X ➡ higher rate coding of type 2X ➡ maximum tetanus of all recruited MUs/fibers within the 70% NA/CNS potential.

Type 1 = 750 total MUs. A maximum of 525 can only be recruited in line with the 70% NA/CNS potential.

Type 2A = 488 total MUs. A maximum of 342 can only be recruited in a maximum effort.

Type 2X = 262 total MUs. A maximum of 183 can only be recruited in a maximum effort.

All combined MUs are listed for the initial rep.

The units of force breakdown for each MU type is noted but not discussed as these diagrams only depict MU activity. Because each MU type has a different unit of force value (1=1, 2A=2, and 2X=3) it can potentially be more confusing when detailing both MU and U. O. F. recruitment and fatigue combined in the same diagram (that is the rationale for the U. O. F. discussion and depiction relative to diagram 3).

BREAKDOWN OF THE MU/FATIGUE PROCESS TO PROVIDE THE REQUIRED AMOUNT OF FORCE. Three categories are listed for each MU type:

Reserve = Total quantity of MUs in the reserve pool before and following each rep. Some are unrecruited and some are previously recruited but not fatigued.

Recruited & Not Fatigued = Total quantity of MUs recruited to assist in the rep but not completely fatigued and still usable.

Recruited & Fatigued = Total quantity of MUs recruited in the rep and completely fatigued at the conclusion of the rep. THE NUMBER IN PARENTHESIS IS THE CUMULATIVE TOTAL OF COMPLETELY FATIGUED MUs OCCURRING SEQUENTIALLY DURING THE SET TO MMF.

The actual rep-by-rep estimate of ATP contribution during each rep is noted (by percentage). Regarding the ATP supplier remember the timelines discussed earlier:

1. Immediate stores @ :03 maximum effort.
2. Creatine Kinase (CK) reaction = ATP ➡ ADP + P + energy and Phosphocreatine (PCr) via CK reaction = Cr and P, with the P added to ADP = new ATP @ :03 to :10-:12 @ maximum effort.
3. Glycolysis (glucose breakdown) @ :12 to 1:40.
4. Aerobic (O2) @ 1:40 and beyond.

Note:

1. Because all energy systems overlap, the intensity of effort determines which one is most heavily relied upon.
2. At any point during an event (either low, moderate, or high intensity) the various possible combinations of the energy system reliance must equal 100%. That is, the ATP energy generated may look something like these:
   - Immediate stores @ 10%, CK reaction @ 85%, Glycolysis @ 4%, and O2 @ 1% or,
   - 95%, 3%, 1.5%, and 0.5%, respectively.

End of rep and time. This will note the recruitment and fatigue status at the start of the first rep (0:00) and completion of each rep at a cadence of :03/rep. This hypothetical is provided to illustrate the timeline of accumulating MU fatigue as reps progress and culminate at the point of MMF.

Total MUs recruited at the start of the event. (i.e., **909** in the 10-RM). The number of MUs recruited to complete further reps are then noted and WILL REMAIN CONSTANT, THEN DECREASE UNTIL FATIGUE PREVENTS MORE FROM BEING RECRUITED. Understand only a certain number will be recruited – no more or no less – to move the resistance depending on its weight. One could consciously recruit more if desired (thus increasing concentric rep velocity) but these examples assume just the minimum number of MUs recruited each rep to move the relative amount of resistance.

Cannot perform a 2nd, 11th, or 36th repetition. This notes the point of the set where the necessary number of MUs cannot be recruited due to complete fatigue and a lack of unfatigued MUs remaining in the reserve pool. Understand there may be a reserve available, but not enough to fully complete another repetition with the given resistance. Even a 1% reduction in the quantity of MUs (and resultant U. O. F.) will preclude the ability to complete another rep. The number of potentially recruitable MUs (unfatigued) for another rep is noted for each MU type, and all of them combined equals the number highlighted in yellow at the bottom of the gray "Total MUs Recruited at the Start..." column.

The total (XXX) at the bottom of the RECRUITED (FATIGUED) column for each MU type lists just that: the total number unavailable because they were used and spent in the completion of the set. Those totals are noted in the summary section.

Total set and repetition time. All examples are depicted using a three second (:03) per repetition velocity to standardize the time-of-exercise element. That is, the elapsed time from the start to finish of each rep will be :03, which will equate to :03 total time in the 1-RM, :30 in the 10-RM, and 1:45 in the 35-RM examples.

Obviously, many time-of-exercise possibilities can exist in the real world. Some trainees may move consciously faster or slower, and some may rest/pause between reps (i.e., slight rest time in a lock-out position). This can vary the total set work time between different individuals. On that, the true time-of-exercise is contingent on these:

1. One's conscious effort to move the resistance relatively fast or slow.

2. The length of each rest/pause taken if they occur (and most likely they will).

3. The number of rest/pause moments taken.

4. Bone (lever) lengths. All other factors being equal, longer levers will make the rep completion lengthier as opposed to shorter levers.

SUMMARY: A recap of the event. The total quantity and percentage of each MU type recruited and completely fatigued and the total of all combined. Also, the amount of contribution of each energy system used to fuel the event is noted.

HYPOTHETICAL MOTOR UNIT (MU) RECRUITMENT, ESTIMATED FATIGUE, AND ENERGY SYSTEM DEMAND FOR AN AVERAGE NEUROLOGICAL ABILITY (70%) AND AVERAGE FIBER TYPE MAKE UP DURING A 1-RM RESISTANCE TRAINING SET

Recruitment process: Type 1 --> max rate coding --> Type 2A --> max rate coding --> Type 2X --> max rate coding

Type	Total	Recruitable @ 70%	Needed for 1st rep	Value	Total	Recruitable @ 70%	Needed for 1st rep
Type 1 - Small, slow to fatigue	750	525	525				
Type 2A - Intermediate	488	342	342				
Type 2X - Large, fast to fatigue	262	183	183				
All combined	1,500	1,050	1,050				

BREAKDOWN OF THE MU RECRUITMENT/FATIGUE PROCESS TO PROVIDE THE REQUIRED AMOUNT OF FORCE TO COMPLETE THE 1-RM:

1-RM

ATP SUPPLIER				END OF REP	TIME	TOTAL MUs RECRUITED AT THE START OF THE 1-RM	T1 FAT	T1 R&NF	T1 RES	T2A FAT	T2A R&NF	T2A RES	T2X FAT	T2X R&NF	T2X RES
Stored	CK	Glyc.	O2			1,050		525	750		342	488		183	262
95%	3%	1.5%	0.5%	1	0:03	958	0	525	750	0	342	488	(92)	91	170
Cannot perform a 2nd repetition				0:04	958	(0)	525	750	(0)	342	488	(92)	91	170

SUMMARY

MOTOR UNITS FATIGUED = 2X = (92)/262 (35%). TOTAL = 6% (92/1,500)
ATP PROVIDED BY (at one point of the set):
Stored = 95%
CK Reaction = 3%
Glycolysis = 1.5%
Aerobic = 0.5%

Diagram 4: Hypothetical MU Recruitment & Fatigue During a 1-RM Event

1-RM NOTES

Because this is an all-out 100% event, all 1,050 recruitable MUs (70% of the 1,500 total) will be recruited at some point in the brief but maximum effort…525 type 1, 342 type 2A, and 183 type 2X.

RESERVE

In this brief maximal effort, a large reserve of MUs will remain. Even though all 1,050 recruitable MUs will be recruited, the max effort fatigues only a partial quantity of the low enduring but strongest 2X group, just enough to prevent a second rep.

RECRUITED & NOT FATIGUED

The vast number of all MUs recruited will have plenty endurance remaining. All recruitable type 1 (525) and 2A (342) will be activated but will not become completely fatigued due to their better endurance as compared to the larger, but lower enduring type 2X (183 total). The :03 total time of the event only affects those 2X MUs, just enough to decrease the reserve pool below the 1,050 needed to continue. During that :03 rep, approximately 35% (91) type 2X remain unfatigued.

RECRUITED & FATIGUED

In this case it is only one rep and done. A second rep is not possible due to the complete fatigue of the low enduring type 2X MUs. All 183 recruitable 2X MUs are recruited and 92 were completely fatigued which leaves the total reserve pool at 958 available (525 type 1 + 342 type 2A + 91 type 2X) at the :04 point/start of a potential second rep. 1,050 total MUs are needed so the remaining pool of 958 will be insufficient. Remember, at any given point only 70% of the maximum total of each type can be recruited even though there is large total in the reserve pool. The depletion of 35% of type 2X is the limiting factor in the 1-RM event.

Regarding the ATP supplier, remember the previously discussed timelines. In this case the 1-RM is completed in a short :03 moment. Also note all energy systems function simultaneously but the intensity of effort dictates which one(s) are relied upon the most, and their total contribution must equal 100%. This extremely intense event is essentially all stored ATP in the muscles (95%), to an extent the CK reaction which is beginning to prime (3%), and negligible glycolysis (1.5%) and oxygen intake (0.5%).

In the end, only 6% of all available MUs/fibers were completely fatigued. From a time-efficiency viewpoint, this shows the ineffectiveness of ultra-heavy training relative to seeking a thorough overload of the greatest quantity of MUs/fibers in a set performed. This is the rationale for using multiple reps (i.e., eight, 12, or 20). They offer a more effective means to thoroughly in-road muscle. More MUs/fibers are repeatedly recruited, more are eventually fatigued, thus "more bang for the buck" is obtained from multiple rep sets performed to MMF as compared to single rep sets.

Diagram 5 depicts the 1-RM event in terms of U. O. F. recruitment and fatigue.

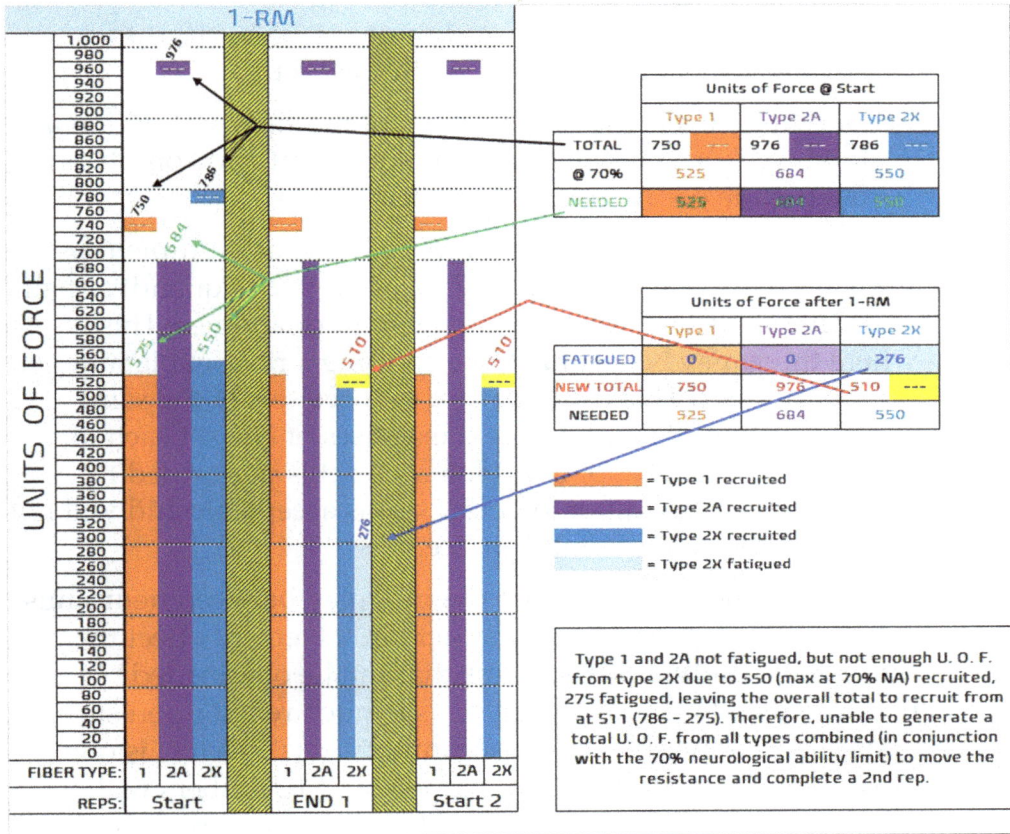

Units of Force @ Start			
	Type 1	Type 2A	Type 2X
TOTAL	750	976	786
@ 70%	525	684	550
NEEDED	525	684	550

Units of Force after 1-RM			
	Type 1	Type 2A	Type 2X
FATIGUED	0	0	276
NEW TOTAL	750	976	510
NEEDED	525	684	550

= Type 1 recruited
= Type 2A recruited
= Type 2X recruited
= Type 2X fatigued

Type 1 and 2A not fatigued, but not enough U. O. F. from type 2X due to 550 (max at 70% NA) recruited, 275 fatigued, leaving the overall total to recruit from at 511 (786 - 275). Therefore, unable to generate a total U. O. F. from all types combined (in conjunction with the 70% neurological ability limit) to move the resistance and complete a 2nd rep.

Diagram 5: Units of Force Recruitment & Fatigue During a 1-RM Event

MORE PRE-DISCUSSION THOUGHTS AND SPECULATION ON MULTIPLE REP SETS TO MMF

1. Recall that on average only 70% of all MUs/fibers one possesses can be recruited in one conscious effort. One who possesses 1,500 total MUs can only "turn on" 1,050 of those at one time, and 30% remain unrecruited and dormant. However, when all is said and done it leaves these questions:

A. Does that mean 30% of all MUs/fibers will not be used regardless of the number of reps completed?

B. Due to the "substitution-rotation" phenomenon, at some point during extended rep sets performed to MMF, will all MUs/fibers be recruited and fatigued 1) from one set only, 2) because many difficult and fatiguing reps are completed, and 3) because one consciously put out 100% effort to achieve that complete MMF on the last rep?

C. Does it take a reasonable number of multiple sets within a total workout session to effectively recruit and completely fatigue the entire spectrum of MUs/fibers?

Over the course of performing multiple sets of multiple reps to MMF it seems likely more than 70% of the entire quantity of all MUs/fibers will be involved at one point or another. This is where there may be a value to performing a reasonable number of multiple sets. This could be two or three sets of the same exercise or two or three different exercises of one set each for the same muscle group. Provided each set is performed to MMF safely, the addition of a few sets is acceptable and will not bring out the "one-set only" police.

2. Regarding question one, does the interplay between neuromuscular recruitment and energy system involvement affect the ultimate quantity of MUs/fibers that can be overloaded? In higher reps sets where glycolysis is a much relied upon supplier of ATP (and metabolite accumulation is a factor) is one fully able to tap into the higher threshold MUs/fibers without the interference from metabolites? (See central vs. peripheral fatigue discussion).

3. In adherence with Henneman's Principle of orderly recruitment and MU/fiber rate coding, does it matter what amount of resistance is used or the number of reps that are performed provided one achieves MMF? That is, is the same quantity of MUs/fibers overloaded regardless if it's a 12-RM or a 20-RM?

4. Knowing high tension elicits the recruitment of the greatest quantity of MUs/fibers, which one is more important...high tension from lower rep/heavier resistance sets (i.e., sets of four to eight reps to MMF) or higher rep/lighter resistance sets (i.e., sets of 10 to 15 reps to MMF)?

5. Regarding the total time to perform each set, a :03 per rep (:015 concentric/up and :015 eccentric/down) is used to illustrate the hypothetical rep time completion and fatigue accumulation to the point of MMF. Realistically, the time of the reps will begin to increase (slower velocity) as fatigue sets in. It's simply due to A) the onset of fatigue and difficulty to continue recruiting MUs/fibers and B) the natural tendency to pause between reps as a result of the fatigue, and as noted, a brief pause allows a tincture of ATP to immediately resynthesize to help the cause. This point clearly reveals that it's mostly about the amount of time muscle is under tension and not simply the number of reps completed.

6. Further, for maximum MU/fiber involvement, is it prudent to perform A) multiple, ultra-heavy, high tension sets (i.e., six or more sets for one to four reps each) which would be less time-efficient or B) a minimal number of lighter resistance, lower initial tension sets that eventually become high-effort near the end point of MMF (i.e., one or two sets for 12 to 16 reps)? The latter would be more time efficient.

7. Because all MUs/fibers will not be recruited initially in multiple rep sets due to submaximal amounts of resistances being used, these questions arise:

   A) Is the total combined recruitment of all three MU/fiber types somewhere in the range of 70% to 85% of the total pool of recruitable MUs/fibers for a relatively lighter 10-RM set, and 50% to 65% of the entire total for an even lighter 35-RM resistance set?

   B) Regarding recruitment of individual MU/fiber types in heavy submaximal and low rep sets to MMF (i.e., 4 to 6) - and due to the demand in compliance with Henneman's Principle and rate coding - is this realistic explanation plausible: 100% of type 1 (first on), 100% of 2A (next on), and 70% to 85% of 2X (last on)?

   C) Alternatively, during a set to MMF with a lighter resistance and higher reps (i.e., 15 to 20), could it be 100% type 1 and 50% to 60% type 2A for the initial reps, then the remainder of MUs/fibers needed to complete the event to MMF provided by the harder-to-recruit type 2X?

D) Logic dictates that the lighter the resistance used, the lower the initial tension will be in all contracting MUs/fibers. That is, a maximum effort 1-RM obviously requires the complete recruitment of all recruitable MU/fiber types, but using 55% of the 1-RM would only require fewer MUs/fibers, less tension, and all depending on one's NA/CNS potential and MU/fiber quantity and distribution. So, over the accumulating reps to MMF with lighter, less initial tension producing resistances, how deep does one recruit into the higher threshold MUs/fibers?

If the amount of resistance was not important to recruit and completely fatigue all recruitable MUs/fibers - and the only necessity was achieving MMF with any amount of resistance - then 40 pounds completed for 88 reps to MMF would be enough to recruit and fatigue all recruitable MUs/fibers. But logic also dictates there is more to the resistance-tension-reps/time relationship and not solely an arbitrary amount of resistance used for max reps to MMF.

E) More specifically, is the amount of resistance that would be considered heavy (i.e., one that would initially activate a high percentage of all MUs/fibers) all that is needed to recruit and completely fatigue all recruitable MUs/fibers provided the set is performed to MMF?

Understand that during any set there may be a high percentage of total MUs/fibers recruited to complete all reps. However, in the end only a minimal quantity of those may have been fatigued and stimulated to adapt to the MMF stress. In example, most resistance training sets will activate the maximum number of low-threshold type 1 MUs/fibers in accordance with Henneman's Principle, but those lower force-generating and higher enduring MUs/fibers will not be stimulated to adapt to the overload stress of the event. The final total quantity of all MUs/fibers stimulated and completely fatigued will therefore be relatively low even though it took 100% effort to complete the task.

HYPOTHETICAL MOTOR UNIT (MU) RECRUITMENT, ESTIMATED FATIGUE, AND ENERGY SYSTEM DEMAND FOR AN AVERAGE NEUROLOGICAL ABILITY (70%) AND AVERAGE FIBER TYPE MAKE UP DURING A 10-RM RESISTANCE TRAINING SET

Recruitment process: Type 1 --> max rate coding --> Type 2A --> max rate coding --> Type 2X --> max rate coding

Type	Motor Units			Units of Force			
	Total	Recruitable @ 70%	Needed for 1st rep	Value	Total	Recruitable @ 70%	Needed for 1st rep
Type 1 - Small, slow to fatigue	750	525	525				
Type 2A - Intermediate	488	342	342				
Type 2X - Large, fast to fatigue	262	183	42				
All combined	1,500	1,050	909				

BREAKDOWN OF THE MU RECRUITMENT/FATIGUE PROCESS TO PROVIDE THE REQUIRED AMOUNT OF FORCE FROM REP 1 THROUGH REP 10:

10-RM

ATP SUPPLIER				END OF REP	TIME	TOTAL MUs RECRUITED AT THE START OF THE 10-RM 909	TYPE 1			TYPE 2A			TYPE 2X		
Stored	CK	Glyc.	O2				RECRUITED & (FATIGUED)	RECRUITED & NOT FATIGUED	RESERVE	RECRUITED & (FATIGUED)	RECRUITED & NOT FATIGUED	RESERVE	RECRUITED & (FATIGUED)	RECRUITED & NOT FATIGUED	RESERVE
					0:00			525	750		342	488		42	262
95%	3%	1.5%	0.5%	1	0:03	909	0	525	750	0	342	488	2	40	260
10%	85%	4%	1%	2	0:06	909	0	525	750	0	342	488	(5) 3	39	257
0%	91%	7%	2%	3	0:09	909	0	525	750	7	335	481	(10) 5	37	252
	80%	18%	2%	4	0:12	909	0	525	750	(21) 14	328	467	(17) 7	35	245
	37%	60%	3%	5	0:15	909	0	525	750	(41) 20	322	447	(26) 9	33	236
	6%	90%	4%	6	0:18	909	0	525	750	(69) 28	314	419	(38) 12	30	224
	0%	95%	5%	7	0:21	909	0	525	750	(124) 55	287	364	(53) 15	27	209
		94%	6%	8	0:24	909	0	525	750	(199) 75	267	289	(71) 18	24	191
		92%	8%	9	0:27	891	0	525	750	(287) 88	201	201	(106) 35	42	156
		91%	9%	10	0:30	861	0	525	750	(387) 100	101	101	(178) 72	63	84
Cannot perform an 11th repetition					0:31	710	(0)	525	750	(387)	101	101	(178)	84	84

MOTOR UNITS FATIGUED = (387)/488 TYPE 2A (79%) and (178)/262 TYPE 2X = 68%). TOTAL = 38% (565/1,500)

SUMMARY

ATP PROVIDED BY (at one point of the set):
Stored = 100%
CK Reaction = 100%
Glycolysis = 95%
Aerobic = 9%

Diagram 6: Hypothetical MU Recruitment & Fatigue During a 10-RM Event

10-RM NOTES

The resistance used for the 10-RM is submaximal, yet relatively heavy compared to zero resistance. That is, the amount of resistance used for 10 reps to MMF can range from 68% to 88% of a 1-RM (contingent on one's NA/CNS potential), which is only 12% to 32% less than maximum. Like the 1-RM, 1,050 MUs are available, but only 909 are needed to complete the first rep because it does not initially require all available. However, as fatigue progresses each rep it will be impossible to recruit the necessary 909 MUs (remember, U.O.F. not factored in here) from the reserve pool and the set will terminate before an 11th rep can be completed.

RESERVE

Because it is a sub-maximal effort not all will be needed initially. The only MUs recruited in the initial rep (time 0:00) are 525 type 1 (70% of 750), 342 intermediate type 2A, and some type 2X (42). Over the set of 10 reps, the demand will increase as fatigue takes its toll and more will be called upon from the reserve pool.

At the end of rep five/0:15 the reserve status is:

- 909 MUs still recruited.
- 525 type 1 still in reserve (unfatigued).
- 447 out of 488 type 2A in reserve.
- 236 out of 262 type 2X in reserve.

As fatigue accumulates to the point where that 11th rep is impossible (at :31) the status is:

- Only 710 MUs are available.
- 525 type 1 still unfatigued.
- 101 type 2A available.
- 84 type 2X available.

RECRUITED & NOT FATIGUED

From reps one to 10, all 525 smaller type 1 MUs will be recruited but not completely fatigued due to their higher endurance capacity. Even tough smaller in size, they contribute to the event because it is a relatively heavy all-out event. The quantity of type 2A MUs recruited and not fatigued will begin to decrease in latter reps because of the greater demand. In example, 289 are recruited in rep nine, but only 88 are fatigued and the remaining 201 are still unfatigued. Type 2X recruitment will begin to increase due to the diminishing 2A reserve pool and the need to continue force output: from 42 (24 + 18) in rep eight to 135 (63 + 72) in rep 10.

RECRUITED & FATIGUED

These are the MUs that have been used during the rep and completely fatigued in the process. The quantity increases as the force output demand increases. The number in parenthesis is the cumulative total of fatigued MUs as such:

Rep 4/0:12 recruited, fatigued, and (cumulative total fatigued):

- Type 1 525 recruited, 0 fatigued, and (0) cumulative total fatigued.
- Type 2A 328, 14, and (21).
- Type 2X 35, 7, and (17).

Rep 9/0:27 recruited, fatigued, and (cumulative total fatigued):

- Type 1 525, 0, and (0).
- Type 2A 201, 88, and (287).
- Type 2X 42, 35, and (106)

At the conclusion of the 10 reps/:30 point there will be an inability to recruit the necessary quantity of MUs to complete an 11th rep. All type 1 MUs will have assisted, may be impaired regarding excitation/coupling ability, but will not be completely fatigued. 387 2A will have been recruited and completely fatigued, and 178 2X will have been used and completely exhausted. The reserve pool will only contain 710 "fresh" MUs, not enough to generate the required units of force to continue the task.

Regarding the ATP supplier remember how energy is supplied. In this case the 10-RM is completed in :30 @ :03/rep. Again, all energy systems function simultaneously but the intensity of effort dictates which one(s) are relied upon the most, and their sums must equal 100%. This submaximal but ultimately intense effort relies on the stored ATP in the muscles (100%), the CK reaction (100%), glycolysis (95%), and some oxygen intake (9%) at various stages of the event.

Here's the "play by play" of the energy supply for the 10-RM event:

- Reps one to two @ :00 to :06 = all stored ATP with the CK reaction increasing.
- Reps two to five @ :06 to :15 = CK reaction declines and glycolysis increasing.
- Reps five to 10 @ :15 to :30 = It's primarily glycolysis here, with oxygen intake revving up, but contributing only minimally.

In the end only 38% of all available MUs were fatigued and thus received an overload stress. From a time-efficiency viewpoint, this again shows the value of multiple reps performed to MMF as compared to a one-and-done 1-RM (6% of all) when seeking a thorough overload of the greatest quantity of MUs per set.

Diagram 7 depicts the 10-RM event in terms of U. O. F. recruitment and fatigue.

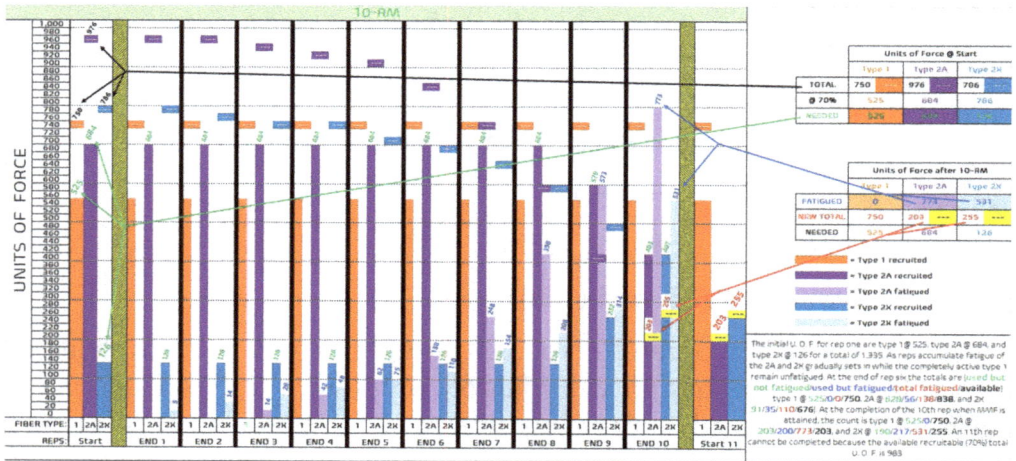

Diagram 7: Units of Force Recruitment & Fatigue During a 10-RM Event

35-RM NOTES

Naturally, the resistance used for a 35-RM event will be much less as compared to the resistance used for the 10-RM. However, due to a greater spectrum of MU recruitment over a lengthier time to reach muscle failure, the lighter resistance can still recruit and fatigue a significant quantity of them.

The amount of resistance used for 35 reps to MMF can vary relative to one's 1-RM. It could range from 46% to 64% of one's maximum. That may seem too light to be considered an effective amount for a resistance training set, but it is still greater than zero resistance. Like any set performed, all MUs are available but in the 35-RM only 769 are needed to complete the initial reps. However, as fatigue progresses on each rep, more MUs will be recruited, and eventually it will be impossible to recruit the necessary MUs. The set will terminate before a 36th rep can be completed.

RESERVE

Due to the sub-maximal effort even fewer MUs will be activated initially. The only MUs recruited in the initial rep (time 0:00) are 525 type 1 (70% of 750) and 244 intermediate type 2A. No type 2X will be needed at the start. Over the entire set of 35 reps the demand will increase

HYPOTHETICAL MOTOR UNIT (MU) RECRUITMENT, ESTIMATED FATIGUE, AND ENERGY SYSTEM DEMAND FOR AN AVERAGE NEUROLOGICAL ABILITY (70%) AND AVERAGE FIBER TYPE MAKE UP DURING A 35-RM RESISTANCE TRAINING SET

Recruitment process: Type 1 --> max rate coding --> Type 2A --> max rate coding --> Type 2X --> max rate coding

Type	Motor Units			Units of Force			
	Total	Recruitable @ 70%	Needed for 1st rep	Value	Total	Recruitable @ 70%	Needed for 1st rep
Type 1 - Small, slow to fatigue	750	525	525	1	750	525	525
Type 2A - Intermediate	488	342	248	2	976	684	496
Type 2X - Large, fast to fatigue	262	183	0	3	786	549	0
All combined	1,500	1,050	773		2,512	1,758	1,021

BREAKDOWN OF THE MU RECRUITMENT/FATIGUE PROCESS TO PROVIDE THE REQUIRED AMOUNT OF FORCE FROM REP 1 THROUGH REP 35:

35-RM

ATP SUPPLIER				END OF REP	TIME	TOTAL MUs RECRUITED AT THE START OF THE 35-RM	TYPE 1			TYPE 2A			TYPE 2X		
Stored	CK	Glyc.	O2				RECRUITED & (FATIGUED)	RECRUITED & NOT FATIGUED	RESERVE	RECRUITED & (FATIGUED)	RECRUITED & NOT FATIGUED	RESERVE	RECRUITED & (FATIGUED)	RECRUITED & NOT FATIGUED	RESERVE
					0:00	769		525	750		244	488		0	262
95%	3%	1.5%	0.5%	1	0:03	769	0	525	750	0	244	488	0	0	262
0%	92%	7%	1%	3	0:09	769	0	525	750	0	244	488	0	0	262
	33%	65%	2%	5	0:15	769	0	525	750	0	244	488	0	0	262
	6%	90%	4%	7	0:21	769	0	525	750	0	244	488	0	0	262
		95%	5%	9	0:27	769	0	525	750	0	244	488	0	0	262
		91%	9%	11	0:33	769	0	525	750	8	236	480	0	0	262
		88%	12%	13	0:39	769	0	525	750	(21) 13	231	467	0	0	262
		85%	15%	15	0:45	769	0	525	750	(40) 19	225	449	0	0	262
		81%	19%	17	0:51	769	0	525	750	(64) 25	219	424	0	0	262
		77%	23%	19	0:57	769	0	525	750	(95) 31	213	393	0	0	262
		73%	27%	21	1:03	769	0	525	750	(134) 39	205	354	0	0	262
		68%	32%	23	1:09	769	0	525	750	(182) 48	196	307	0	0	262
		63%	37%	25	1:15	769	0	525	750	(240) 59	185	248	0	0	262
		57%	43%	27	1:21	769	0	525	750	(306) 66	178	183	0	0	262
		51%	49%	29	1:27	746	0	525	750	(387) 82	98	101	10	31	252
		45%	55%	31	1:33	719	0	525	750	(488) 98	0	0	(31) 21	75	231
		39%	61%	33	1:39	687	0	525	750	0	0	0	(63) 32	130	199
		32%	68%	35	1:45	678	0	525	750	0	0	0	(109) 45	108	153
Cannot perform a 36th repetition					1:46	633	(0)	525	750	(488)	0	0	(109)	108	153

SUMMARY

MOTOR UNITS FATIGUED = (488)/488 2A (100%) and (109)/262 2X (42%). **TOTAL = 40% (597)/1,500**
ATP PROVIDED BY (at one point of the set):
Stored = 100%
CK Reaction = 100%
Glycolysis = 95%
Aerobic = 68%

Diagram 8: Hypothetical MU Recruitment & Fatigue During a 35-RM Event

as fatigue takes its toll, and again more will be called upon from the reserve pool.

At the end of rep 15/0:45 the reserve status is:

- 769 MUs still recruited.

- 525 type 1 still in reserve (unfatigued).

- 449 out of 488 type 2A in reserve.

- All 262 type 2X in reserve.

At the end of rep 29/1:27 the reserve status is:

- 746 MUs still recruited.

- 525 type 1 still in reserve (unfatigued).

- 101 out of 488 type 2A in reserve.

- 252 type 2X in reserve (at this point they will now be re-cruited due to the complete depletion of the 2A reserve pool that will occur during the 31st rep).

As fatigue accumulates to the point where that 36th rep is impossible (at 1:46) the status is:

- Only 633 MUs are available.

- 525 type 1 still completely unfatigued.

- 0 type 2A available.

- 108 type 2X available.

RECRUITED & NOT FATIGUED

From rep one to 35 all 525 smaller type 1 MUs will be recruited but will not completely fatigue due to their higher endurance capacity. Like the 10-RM, they are required in accordance with Henneman's Principle, and as the demand of the event becomes more intense they will still be needed to assist nearing the point of MMF. The number of type 2A MUs recruited and not fatigued will begin to decrease in latter reps because of the greater demand: 244 (178 + 66) following rep 27 to 180 (98 + 82) following rep 29. The type 2X will begin to assist during the 29th rep (41 = 31 + 10) due to the diminishing 2A reserve pool and the need to continue force output, then rise to complete the 33rd rep (162=130+32) but drop during the 35th rep (153=108+45).

RECRUITED & FATIGUED

The lengthier 35-RM event will gradually diminish the entire pool of 2A MUs and some 2X. The number in parenthesis is the cumulative total of completely fatigued MUs as such:

Rep 17/0:51 recruited, fatigued, and (cumulative total fatigued):

- Type 1 525, 0, and (0).
- Type 2A 219, 25, and (64).
- Type 2X 262, 0, and (0).

Rep 33/1:39 recruited, fatigued, and (cumulative total fatigued):

- Type 1 525, 0, and (0).
- Type 2A 0, 0, and (0).
- Type 2X 130, 32, and (63).

At the conclusion of the 35 reps/1:45 there will be an inability to recruit the necessary quantity of MUs to complete a 36th rep. All type 1 MUs will have assisted (but will not be fatigued), all 488 2A will have been recruited and completely fatigued, and 109 2X will have been used and completely exhausted. The reserve pool will only contain 633 "fresh" MUs, not enough to generate the required units of force to continue the task.

Regarding ATP suppliers and the longer duration 1:45 @ :03/rep timeline, after immediate stores (100%) and the CK reaction (100%) are fully tapped, it digs largely into glycolysis (95%) and involves more oxygen intake (68%) compared to the 1- and 10-RM examples. This has greater implications regarding the value of higher rep sets that can be used for circuit training and other energy-depleting resistance programs. Because they create a high metabolic effect via an increased muscle demand, a sustained heart rate, and an overall greater energy depletion (ATP during and post-exercise), higher rep sets have a place in fat-loss and/or cardiorespiratory-enhancing programs in as much as they contribute to that goal provided proper nutritional intake is addressed.

Here's the "play by play" of the energy supply for the 35-RM event:

- Reps one to three @ :00 to :09 = all stored ATP with the CK reaction replenishing immediate ATP.
- Reps three to seven @ :09 to :21 = The CK reaction comes to a screeching halt and glycolysis is now stepping up.

- Reps seven to 35 @ :21 to 1:45 = glycolysis is now running the show, but at the 1:00 point oxygen intake begins to make a greater contribution as more time has been allowed for ATP to be generated aerobically via the mitochondrial process.

Diagram 9 depicts the 35-RM event in terms of U. O. F. recruitment and fatigue.

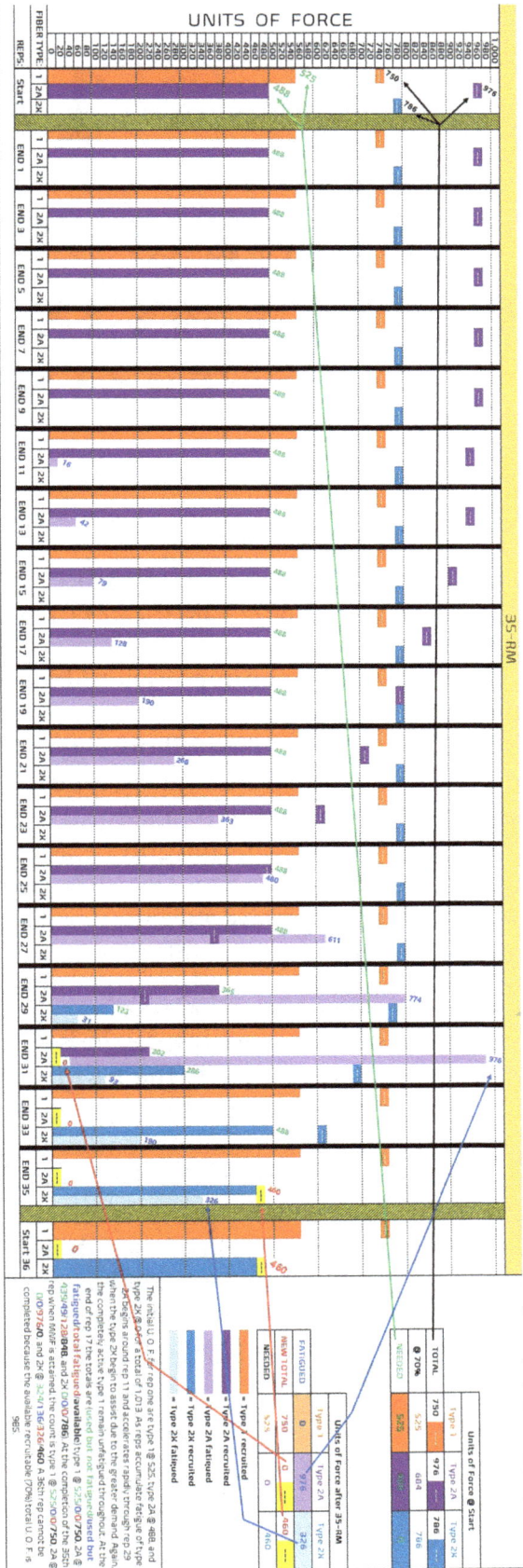

ram 9: Units of Force Recruitment & Fatigue During a 35-RM Event

11

ANSWERS TO COMMON QUESTIONS IN RESISTANCE TRAINING

HOW ARE MUSCLES ACTIVATED DURING A ONE REP MAXIMUM (1-RM) COMPARED TO A 35-RM?

As depicted in the hypothetical MU recruitment diagrams, the heavier resistance used in a 1-RM recruits a maximum quantity of MUs during the very brief but 100% all-out event. Because of this, a portion of the much needed but less enduring type 2X MUs will be completely fatigued and unable to assist with a second rep. That is the nature of a 1-RM: a very short event, the fatigue of a significant quantity of the higher threshold and larger type 2X MUs, and the reliance on the immediate ATP stores. But because it fatigues just enough of the much needed 2X MUs, it's done. There is minimal use of the glycolytic system, hence no build-up of pain-inducing metabolites.

The resistance used for the 35-RM by necessity will be much lighter than the resistance used in the 1-RM. Initially, fewer MUs will be needed to move the resistance through the range of motion repetitively. As fatigue begins to set in and render the heavily recruited type 2A MUs useless, the higher threshold type 2X MUs will be recruited to complete the task. Eventually, peripheral fatigue will shut down the event following the 35th rep, just enough to leave the trainee without enough recruitable units of force available to complete that 36th rep even though a reserve is still available (all type 1 and approximately 60% of type 2X). In contrast to the 1-RM, the lengthier 35-RM creates more havoc in the recruited MUs due to the greater work involved and more metabolite accumulation from the more depended upon glycolytic system.

WHAT ENERGY SYSTEM(S) FUEL THE VARIOUS NUMBER OF REPS THAT CAN BE PERFORMED?

Depending on the time under tension/rep velocity and cadence, a lower number of reps performed (one to five/:03 to :15) uses immediate stores of ATP and the resynthesis of ATP via the CK reaction. A moderate number of reps performed (five to 20/:15 to 1:00) uses immediate stores, the CK reaction, and a large contribution of glycolysis. A higher number of reps performed (20 to 40/1:00 to 2:00) uses immediate, CK reaction, glycolysis full-throttle, and the aerobic system to assist as the number of reps go even higher.

Knowing how the energy systems fuel resistance training can facilitate better program design in terms of rep prescriptions, recovery time between sets, total workout volume, and assuring adequate between-session recovery time is scheduled.

WHY DO TWO PEOPLE WITH THE SAME BODY TYPE AND 1-RM DIFFER IN THE NUMBER OF REPS PERFORMED TO MMF WITH THE SAME PERCENTAGE OF THE 1-RM (I.E., 10 REPS VS. 12 REPS WITH 80%)?

That genetic factor is the primary reason, mainly one's MU/fiber type quantity and distribution combined with their NA/CNS potential. Here are two examples: 1) two people with the same 1-RM, body types, and skeletal leverage and 2) two people with different 1-RMs and skeletal leverages, but similar body types:

1. **Same 1-RM** = 200 lbs./91 kgs. and 80% = 160 lbs./73 kgs.

   Person 1: 10 reps with 80% of the 1-RM.

   Person 2: 12 reps with 80% of the 1-RM.

Same 1-RM explanation

   Person 1 - Average NA/CNS potential + average MU/fiber type quantity and distribution of all types = average ability for 10 reps with 80% of the 1-RM.

   Person 2 - **Above average** NA/CNS potential + **below average** quantity of the stronger 2X, average type 1, and **above average** 2A. They can recruit more MUs/fibers in the 1-RM, but they have fewer stronger 2X, so it averages out and equals person 1. Their ability to perform more reps with the 80% of the 1-RM is due to the **above average** quantity of 2A which slightly trumps their **above average** NA/CNS potential that offers less of a reserve.

2. Different 1-RMs.

Person 3: 250 lbs./114 kgs. and 80% = 200 lbs./91 kgs.

13 reps with 80% of the 1-RM.

Person 4: 315 lbs./143 kgs. and 80% = 252 lbs./114 kgs.

9 reps with 80% of the 1-RM.

Different 1-RMs explanation

Person 3 – Average skeletal leverage + **below average** NA/CNS potential + **above average** quantity of type 1, **below average** 2A, and average 2X MUs/fibers. They can recruit fewer MUs/fibers in a 1-RM but have a greater reserve pool. Their combined type 1 (**above average**) and 2A (**below average**) slightly lowers their endurance potential, but their greater reserve pool trumps that, thus the ability to complete 13 reps with 80% of the 1-RM.

Person 4 – **Above average** skeletal leverage + **above average** NA/CNS potential + **below average** type 1, **above average** type 2A, and average 2X MUs/fibers. They are exceptionally strong due skeletal leverage, NA/CNS potential, and the combined **slight above average** quantity of the stronger 2A (**above average**) and 2X (average) MUs/fibers. Their inability to perform as many reps with 80% of the 1-RM as compared to person 3 is due to their **above average** NA/CNS potential (lower reserve pool) and the combined type 1 (**below average**) and 2A (**above average**) MUs/fibers equating to only **slightly above average endurance potential**.

IS THE QUANTITY OF MUS/FIBERS RECRUITED AND FATIGUED IN ANY SET TO MMF SIMILAR REGARDLESS OF THE AMOUNT OF RESISTANCE USED AND NUMBER OF REPS COMPLETED (I.E., LIGHT RESISTANCE X 20 REPS VS. HEAVY RESISTANCE X EIGHT REPS)?

Even though that question was presented in the pre-discussion thoughts and speculation on the 1-RM and 35-RM multiple rep sets, the answer is most likely no. As can be seen in the 1-RM, 10-RM, and 35-RM diagrams, the end results reveal the approximate quantities of each type completely fatigued. It's largely dependent on 1) the amount of resistance used (dictating the tension created at the start of the set) and the number of reps performed/time to MMF.

On a continuum with a 1-RM on one end and the 35-RM on the other, the ultra-heavy, higher tension-creating 1-RM involves all recruitable MUs/fibers but only fatigues a small portion of the them... the larger, stronger, but less-enduring type 2X. The 35-RM creates less tension initially (i.e., fewer MUs/fibers required), but due to the length of the event (i.e., 1:45) more MUs/fibers are involved as reps and fatigue accumulate to the 35th rep. All weaker and smaller type 1 are recruited but not fatigued (but may experience temporary excitation/coupling impairment), the reserve pool of intermediate type 2A is completely fatigued, and only a partial recruitment and fatigue of the not-initially-recruited 2X MUs/fibers occurs due to the less initial tension created, but their need during the latter demanding reps.

WHY IS ONE ABLE TO PERFORM ADDITIONAL REPS FOLLOWING BRIEF PAUSES DURING A SET, USUALLY HOLDING THE RESISTANCE IN THE LOCKED-OUT/INITIAL STARTING POINT OF AN EXERCISE?

It all comes down to time under tension and the ability to resynthesize ATP. Recall ATP is broken down to release energy for muscle contraction through the process of hydrolysis as follows: ATP ➡ energy + ADP+P. It is resynthesized via the creatine kinase (CK) reaction as follows: ADP + P ➡ CK reaction @ add P (from creatine phosphate [CP]) + ADP = new ATP. So, how does this happen during a set?

A constant tension on the muscle(s) (i.e., no resting) means ATP must be continually shuttled to the sites where it is needed to maintain actin-myosin cross-bridging. When a trainee pauses/rests in the locked-out position, it usually occurs because they are experiencing fatigue and seek a brief respite. For example, in a demanding set of 15 reps to muscle fatigue one may instinctively feel the need to briefly lock-out/pause when double digit reps (at 11 or 12) occur because those working muscles are becoming fatigued. That brief rest/pause lessens the muscle tension just enough to allow the CK reaction to resynthesize ADP + P back to a few more molecules of ATP that can be used to squeeze out an additional rep or two. Not much is resynthesized due to the minimal amount of time available, but it can be just enough to shuttle more ATP to the actin/myosin binding sites until it is impossible to provide any more to complete the task (in this case, a 16th rep).

As mentioned in the energy systems discussion, assuring an adequate supply of intramuscular creatine phosphate – either through diet or supplementation – allows for a few additional seconds of force output near the end of difficult sets performed to MMF.

WHAT CAUSES MUSCLE FAILURE IN ANY SET REGARDLESS IF LOW REPS OR HIGH REPS ARE COMPLETED?

It could be a lack of ATP, impairment of the actin-myosin cross-bridging, and/or calcium ion overload/disruption. More specifically, lower-rep sets (i.e., under :15) deplete immediate stores of ATP, then rely on the CK reaction to briefly resynthesize new ATP before that system fails. In higher rep sets it could be either the immediate depletion of ATP, the inability to resynthesize ATP, and/or the disruption of cross-bridging due to peripheral fatigue resulting from metabolite accumulation from the process of ATP generated by glycolysis. Bottom line: with no ATP available to produce actin-myosin cross-bridging, no more force can be produced, and the event terminates.

That is the reason why higher rep sets to MMF are more discomforting than lower rep sets to MMF. In plain English, it takes more intestinal fortitude to grind out sets of 15 to 25+ reps via glycolysis and the inevitable discomfort of muscle acidity that comes with it as compared to heavier, lower rep, and shorter time under tension sets that cease due to quicker fatigue of the immediate ATP-dependent type 2X MUs/fibers. No discomforting metabolite accumulation occurs in those heavier, short term events.

IS THERE A VALUE TO PERFORMING SINGLE JOINT EXERCISES AS OPPOSED TO MULTI-JOINT EXERCISES DUE TO MU/FIBER DIFFERENCES BETWEEN MUSCLE GROUPS?

A single joint exercise (i.e., chest fly) involves only the shoulder joint (but more than one muscle group). A multi-joint exercise (i.e., chest press) involves the shoulder joint along with the elbow joint, therefore adding the elbow extensors to the mix. The greater the number of muscle groups involved, the greater the potential to have disparities between muscle group contributions and skeletal leverage configurations.

With a chest fly it's mostly about the MU/fiber type, quantity, and distribution in the pectorals and anterior deltoids to move the upper arm through the exercise range of motion. The only "weak link" so to say would be any unfavorable fiber type, quantity, and/or distribution in either of those muscles. Because the chest press requires the addition of the triceps - and consequently a second joint involvement - it's now contingent on the MU/fiber type and quantity in that muscle group. If the tricep MU/fiber type and quantity is unfavorable, it would be the weak link and limit the amount of overload stress placed on the more favorable pectorals and anterior deltoids, as explained in the breakdown below.

A combined average strength in pectorals, **above average** strength in the anterior deltoids, and **below average** strength in the triceps would be:

- Pectorals = average type 1, **below average** 2A, and **above average** 2X.

- Anterior deltoid = **below average** type 1, **above average** 2A, and average 2X.

- Triceps = **above average** type 1, average 2A, and **below average** 2X.

The chest press results will be limited by the weaker triceps, thus the quality of overload on the pectorals and anterior deltoids will be diminished. In this case, a single joint chest fly may be more beneficial to better target those muscles. A separate tricep exercise could then be used to maximally target them using a more relevant resistance and rep scheme.

Not to discount the value of multi-joint exercises, in some cases it's prudent to add single joint exercises (i.e., lateral raise, bent-over fly, leg extension, hip extension) to better target single muscles that would normally be limited by smaller/weaker muscles involved in a multi-joint exercise.

WHY ARE SOME PEOPLE FREAKISHLY STRONG WHILE OTHERS ARE UNFORTUNATELY VERY WEAK?

Genetics, of course. We've all seen it: some "doesn't-look-the part" person bench presses or squats a way above average amount of resistance. If you haven't figured it out by now, the reason behind such unusual performances is their genetic endowment. Not to discount their hard work and training consistency, those freakishly strong humans are blessed with raw talent: it could be above average skeletal leverage, an above average quantity of the larger and stronger type 2X MU/fibers distributed in the relevant muscles, and/or the distinct advantage of being able to recruit an above average quantity of those MUs/fibers in the particular event. Some possess one or two of those while the super genetic freaks may possess all those characteristics. And because they are who they are, they're usually disciplined with their diet, highly skilled, and motivated to perform well.

On the flip side are the genetically less endowed. Empathy for them, but they can still maximize whatever potential they possess through hard, consistent, and intelligent training.

SHOULD ALL SETS BE PERFORMED TO MOMENTARY MUSCLE FATIGUE?

Momentary muscle fatigue (MMF) – the inability to SAFELY perform further reps due to a disruption in the contractile process – is objective. When one "Hits the wall" or "Gives 100% effort" it is measurable. Not performing sets to MMF can work, but it then becomes a subjective gray area. When should a person stop…two reps prior to MMF? Four reps? Rather than leave it to chance, it makes sense to complete sets with 100% effort to avoid that confusion.

Whatever 100% is that day, give it and record it. Record the exact number of reps completed, but do not include partner assisted reps. One will then know exactly what to document and what the goal for the forthcoming session will be. Yes, gutting out those hard-to-get reps is discomforting, but think about it: if you do it on your own volition you were capable of it in the first place. If you don't do it knowing you could have, it was not a 100% effort. Sets performed to MMF safely leaves no doubt that an overload was created that can accurately be recorded for future reference.

If one is just beginning a training program or they're soft and cannot deal with the temporary discomfort that comes with grinding out hard-to-get reps, know this: whether a set is performed for six reps or 20 reps, the last few are the key to eliciting a training effect (21). In example, during a heavy set of six reps, the last two create that maximum overload stimulus. Similarly, in a lighter set of 20 reps, reps 16 through 20 do the same. On the surface that contradicts the recommendation to train to MMF. It does, but it's better than doing nothing when initially learning to train properly. Over time, though, there comes a time when one needs to tolerate temporary discomfort to make further gains, so learn to become comfortable with being uncomfortable. Spend those few additional seconds (literally) performing those last hard-to-get but attainable reps. Grow a pair and do it.

Training to MMF is also more time efficient. For the most part exuding a high intensity of effort means fewer sets are required to elicit an objective training stimulus. That means less time spent training.

There is a limit to how many sets are either reasonable or unnecessary overkill. Performing too many eventually becomes unnecessary, subjective, and may disrupt proper recovery time. Hence, for a proper dose of muscle stimuli and objective documentation of all exercises, sets, and reps, think quality vs. quantity. The underpinning of a sensible progressive training program should be train hard and by necessity train briefly, and do it as safely as possible.

WHAT NUMBER OF REPS ARE MOST EFFECTIVE FOR INCREASING 1) STRENGTH, 2) POWER, 3) LOCAL MUSCLE ENDURANCE, AND 4) MUSCLE SIZE?

There are no cut-and-dried specific number of reps to perform for any of those pursuits. The largest influence are the many genetic differences among people, especially the type and quantity of MUs/fibers in the targeted muscle(s) and the NA/CNS potential factor (average, below average, or above average). On those alone there are a multitude of possible outcomes as were covered in the 10-RM and 35-RM discussions. Therefore, a one-size-fits-all approach does not work, and it should be individualized as much as possible. Specific reps to MMF tests and data from prior training documentation can be used to determine the optimal number of reps to use for one's specific goals.

Two Discussions That May Simplify The Optimal Number Of Reps To Perform

1. *Relationship between strength, power, and local muscular endurance.*

   It stands to reason that increasing muscle strength also increases the ability to express increased power and local muscle endurance. Because progressive resistance training enables one to recruit a greater amount of their inherent total MU/fiber quantity, they will:

   A) Possess the ability to recruit those additional MUs/fibers consciously faster in any given effort (improved power).

B) Possess a greater reserve of unfatigued MUs/fibers (independent of their NA/CNS potential) that can be used to perform more reps with submaximal resistances (improved local muscle endurance).

Regarding power, it's formula is power = force x distance/time. Greater force (strength) applied over a given distance (exercise range, or any athletic skill limb movement distance) in the least amount of time results in a greater power output. The velocity of the time factor is essentially improved through the specific practice of the exact movements or skills needed (see Principle of Specificity discussion).

In resistance training exercises, recall it's impossible to move a heavy resistance relatively fast (law of gravity, thank you Sir Isaac Newton). The only logical means to move any resistance faster is to either lighten the load of the object or become stronger. It's impossible to throw an over-weight baseball (i.e., two pounds/32.0 ounces) faster than a regulation weight baseball (i.e., between 5.0 and 5.25 ounces/142 and 149 grams) assuming maximum effort is applied with each. And the heavier the object becomes, the slower the velocity it will possess, all other factors being equal.

If one has improved their strength and now has more MUs/fibers to tap into, they could throw the over-weight baseball with a faster velocity as compared to the velocity thrown when they were weaker.

Regarding local muscular endurance, refer to the prior examples of resistance used/reps achieved in initial workouts compared to those used in workouts following 60 days of training. In example, on day one a person may possess a 1-RM of 200 lbs./91 kgs. and the ability to lift 160 lbs./73 kgs. for a 10-RM. On day 60 following a progressive resistance training program and now possessing a 1-RM of 225 lbs./102 kgs. (stronger), they will be able to perform more than 10 reps to MMF with 160 lbs./73 kgs. Again, the relationship between muscle strength and local muscle endurance is undisputable.

2. *Determining the optimal rep range for different muscle groups.*

Because increased muscle strength not only improves 1-RM ability, it also improves the ability to generate greater power output and the ability to perform more reps with submaximal resistances. So, what are the optimal number of reps one should perform?

Because of different abilities among the population in both the quantity and distribution of MUs/fibers and NA/CNS potential, there is likely an optimal range of reps one should perform that will maximally recruit and fatigue the greatest quantity of MUs/fibers they possess. And this range of reps not only differs between everyone, it likely differs between the muscle groups of each person. Therefore, it's prudent to determine specific rep ranges for all major muscle groups based on their estimated genetic endowment. This can be accomplished by either 1) trial and error/prior experience or 2) various resistance tests that involve testing for a 1-RM and specific percentages of the 1-RM performed to MMF.

A) Trial and error/prior experience.

Most veteran trainees with years of training experience can usually determine what works best for them. A mixture of workouts that involve lower, moderate, and higher reps will assure muscle tissue is exposed to different stress loads, independent of one's MU/fiber type quantity and distribution and NA/CNS potential. Remember, any progressive resistance training program that enhances force output potential will allow better expressions of maximum force (strength), quick force (power), and force needed for an extended time (local muscle endurance).

If one desires to focus more on one type force expression, they can use a specific range of reps for that purpose. One veteran trainee may have determined using three to six reps work best for them regarding improving pure strength for the front torso pushing muscles (i.e., chest, incline, and overhead presses) while another determined better results were achieved with six to 10 reps. Likewise, one who wants to focus more on local muscle endurance may have determined reps in the 15 to 20 range are best, while another person favors a 20 to 25 range of reps.

Whatever the case, the more resistance training experience one has the better they can determine what best suits them.

B) 1-RM/maximum rep tests.

If one wants to get more specific and better determine an ideal number of reps to complete, they can perform specific tests to estimate their approximate MU/fiber quantity and distribution and NA/CNS potential for specific muscle groups/exercises. This involves the performance of a 1-RM and subsequent sets to MMF with submaximal resistances of the 1-RM.

The 1-RM reveals maximum force output ability displayed mostly by the type 2X and partly by type 2A quantity and distribution in the acting muscles. It's a brief, 100% effort that relies on stored ATP in those MUs/fibers. If the result is extraordinarily high, it likely indicates an above average quantity of 2X MUs/fibers (and to an extent 2A) independent of body type and skeletal leverage. It could also be a result of an above average NA/CNS potential that allows them to recruit more total MUs/fibers than the average person, including more of the stronger type 2X. Body type and skeletal leverage are not force-generating, thus are only constant variables relative to each person's ability and are irrelevant in the pursuit of the ideal rep numbers for different muscle groups.

Another reason why these tests may offer insight into predicting ability and assigning specific reps is due to the forgotten factor of energy system involvement to produce ATP. In review of energy system supply of ATP, aside from the immediate stores that fuel the 1-RM, recall the quick resynthesis of ATP via the creatine kinase reaction during intense sets lasts from :03 to :15. That amount of time would equate to the completion of approximately one to six reps (depending on the rep velocity and cadence) and rely on those fast-to-fatigue higher threshold type 2X MUs/fibers.

Glycolysis begins to supply more ATP as reps extend beyond :15 up to 1:30. This would equate to reps in the range of seven to around 30, again depending on rep velocity and cadence. This timeline would significantly rely on the intermediate type 2A MUs/fibers as they are both strong and enduring.

Performing a heavy set to MMF – then taking a brief recovery – and repeating that set would be a reasonable test to estimate high-threshold type 2X MU/fiber quantity. Performing a moderately heavy set to MMF fatigue in the same manner - but resting a few seconds longer – could estimate the quantity of the intermediate type 2A MUs/fibers.

When attempting to estimate NA/CNS potential it becomes more subjective. However, similar tests performed to MMF may offer more insight into one's NA/CNS potential in conjunction with the estimated MU/fiber type quantities. It's not an exact science but it may reveal odd disparities between one's 1-RM performance and reps achieved with various percentages of it, either average, below average, or above average.

GUIDELINES FOR TESTING MU/FIBER TYPES AND NA/CNS POTENTIAL

1. Establish a 1-RM on designated exercises. Assure safety by using a competent training partner/spotter to assist and supervise.

2. Use proper exercise form on all sets: control the resistance, work through a complete range of motion, and do not count partner/spotter-assisted reps.

3. Record all test results: the amount of resistance used and the number of reps completed to momentary muscle fatigue.

4. Due to multiple tests performed to MMF for different muscle groups (1-RM, MU/fiber type, and if desired the NA/CNS tests), testing must be logically scheduled over several days for best approximations. Fatigue accumulation from multiple tests to MMF on a single day will interfere with accuracy. Use a seven to 10-day period to conduct all tests to assure accuracy. Examples:

Day 1 (Monday)

Perform a 1-RM test on three different exercises: an upper body pull (i.e., pulldown), lower body multi-joint leg push (i.e., leg press), and upper body push (i.e., chest press).

Perform one MU/fiber type (i.e., 2X) or one NA/CNS max rep

test for those exercises. Assure ample recovery time following the 1-RM tests and between each max rep test. A 5:00 recovery time between any test is necessary.

Day 2 or 3 (Tuesday or Wednesday)

Perform a different pull (i.e., seated row), leg (i.e., dead lift), and push (i.e., overhead press) 1-RM test. If not, a MU/fiber type and/or NA/CNS max rep test can be completed for those 1-RM test exercises that were completed on day one. Again, to assure best results use at least 5:00 recovery time between any test.

Day 4 or 5 (Thursday or Friday)

Perform some combination of two or three different exercise tests for a 1-RM, MU/fiber type, and/or NA/CNS ability with ample recovery time between each.

Example:

Bent-over row 1-RM test. (rest 5:00)

Chest press NA/CNS max rep test. (rest 5:00)

Squat 1-RM test. (rest 5:00)

Pulldown 2X max rep test. (rest 5:00)

Leg curl 1-RM test.

Day 6 or 7 (Saturday or Sunday)

Same as day 4 or 5 but use different exercises.

TEST FOR 2X MU/FIBER TYPE

1. Use 90% of a 1-RM for max reps (should range from 1 to 5). This assures maximum fatigue of the type 2X MUs/fibers.

2. Rest exactly :30. The :30 begins when the resistance is racked/disengaged. When :30 elapses, the resistance must immediately be engaged and moving in the second set.

3. Repeat for max reps. If the result is:

   > 75% of the number of 1st set reps = below average quantity of 2X.

50% of the number of 1ˢᵗ set reps = average quantity of 2X.

< 25% of the number of 1ˢᵗ set reps = above average quantity of 2X.

Rationale: Of the three MU/fiber types, the quantity and distribution of 2X is critical for maximum strength. Although all three types are recruited in a 1-RM, it is the quantity of 2X that distinguishes strength differences from one to another. All other factors being equal, one who possesses more 2X – thus possessing more units of force - will exhibit greater strength.

The 90% resistance for max reps will take from :03 to :15. During this 100% effort a maximum quantity of the strongest (but low-enduring) 2X MUs/fibers will be recruited and fatigued. The :30 rest between sets allows for approximately 50% recovery and replenishment of ATP in the fatigued 2X MUs/fibers. Therefore, when the second set is performed for max reps, one's approximate quantity and distribution of the 2X MUs/fibers in the working muscles can be approximated by the results obtained in step three above:

> 75% of the number of 1ˢᵗ set reps (i.e., 1ˢᵗ set = 5 reps; 2ⁿᵈ set = 4 reps). This means one is relatively weaker, has a below average quantity of 2X, and has more type 2A. Only a minimal number of the lower quantity of type 2X MUs/fibers that were recruited and fatigued were able to recover and contribute to the 2ⁿᵈ set. This put more emphasis on the more enduring intermediate 2A MUs/fibers.

50% of the number of 1ˢᵗ set reps (i.e., 1ˢᵗ set = 4 reps; 2ⁿᵈ set = 2 reps). Probably average strength and an average quantity of 2X MUs/fibers. Approximately one-half of them were able to contribute to the 2ⁿᵈ set.

< 25% of the number of 1ˢᵗ set reps (i.e., 1ˢᵗ set = 3 reps; 2ⁿᵈ set = 0 reps). An above average quantity of 2X. This person's 1-RM is relatively heavy due to this, but because many 2X were recruited and fatigued in set one they were unable to recover following the :30. The relative lower quantity of 2A (and type 1) were unable generate enough U. O. F. to complete additional reps.

TEST FOR 2A MU/FIBER TYPE:

The quantity and distribution of 2A MUs/fiber types can to an extent be gleaned from the type 2X test result. The ability to perform 90% of a 1-RM for 75% of the 1ˢᵗ set reps indicates below average 2X, but most likely either an average or above average quantity and distribution of

2A (especially if one is relatively strong). However, a similar specific max rep test can be performed exclusively for the intermediate 2A type MUs/fibers as follows:

1. 70% of a 1-RM for max reps (approximately 8 to 25). This will recruit and fatigue a large quantity of 2A MUs/fibers due to the duration of the event (:25 to :50+).

2. Rest exactly :45. The :45 begins when the resistance is racked/ disengaged. When :45 elapses, the resistance must immediately be engaged and movng in the second set.

3. Repeat for max reps. If the result is:

> 80% of the number of 1st set reps = above average quantity of 2A.

60% of the number of 1st set reps = average quantity of 2A.

< 40% of the number of 1st set reps = below average quantity of 2A.

Rationale: The longer duration of the event will call into play the full extent of the recruitable 2A MUs/fibers. They will be highly depended upon with assistance from some 2X that will also be recruited and fatigued. The accumulation of more fatiguing type 2A and some 2X will significantly tap into the 2A reserve pool as the reps accumulate and glycolysis ramps up past six reps/:18, all the way to 15 to 20+ reps/ :45+.

Again, all MU/fiber types will be involved: from the lower force type 1 which are not fatiguing due to their high endurance capacity, to the highly depended on 2A grinding out maximum reps, to the highest threshold type 2X. Remember, the significantly heavy 70% of a 1-RM resistance is capable of activating many MUs/fibers.

There will be more metabolic waste production that will need to be metabolized (i.e., Ca+, lactate, hydrogen ions) so peripheral fatigue is an issue. The :45 recovery time allows for approximately 60 to 65% of depleted ATP to be replenished in the fatigued fibers. Therefore…

> 80% of the number of 1st set reps (i.e., 1st set = 20 reps; 2nd set = 16 reps). This indicates the probability of an above average quantity of 2A MUs/fibers. This person is most likely a bit weaker (less 2X) and possesses an average quantity and distribution of type 1. Many of the large quantity of 2A MUs/fibers recruited and fatigued and were able to recover contribute to the 2nd set. The small quantity of type 2X did not

offer as much assistance and the more enduring type 1 MUs/fibers always assist which many seem to forget (Henneman's Principle).

55% - 60% of the number of 1st set reps (i.e., 1st set = 15 reps; 2nd set = 8 or 9 reps). Probably an average quantity of 2A MUs/fibers. Slightly over one half of them were able to contribute to the 2nd set.

< 40% of the number of 1st set reps (i.e., 1st set = 18 reps; 2nd set = 7 reps). Probably a below average quantity of 2A. This person's 1-RM may be relatively heavy if they possess an above average quantity and distribution of 2X MUs/fibers, but the lower quantity of 2A are not enough to perform many reps in set two. Fewer will be available to generate enough units of force, even with the assistance of an average quantity and distribution of the smaller, weaker, but more enduring type 1 MUs/fibers.

RELATIVE STRENGTH SCORE AND TESTING FOR NA/CNS POTENTIAL:

Naturally, if a person possesses a muscular and lean body it is assumed they are relatively strong. Also, the more body mass one has, the greater the total quantity of MUs/fibers they possess thus the greater their strength potential. On the other hand, if they lack muscle – or possess more body fat mass – most likely they are relatively weaker. Therefore, it stands to reason a larger body with more functional muscle mass (lower body fat percentage) can display greater force output as compared to one with a similar or smaller body type but with less functional muscle mass (higher body fat percentage = less relative muscle).

But what about the exceptionally strong person with an average build and no evidence of prior training? Most have seen that person in the gym…looks normal, seemingly little athletic ability, no exceptional muscle mass, etc., but can bench press or squat an exceptional amount of resistance. Similarly, there's that person who looks like a badass but displays results analogous to a person on a hunger strike. In any of those cases, their ability is likely dictated by an above or below average NA/CNS potential.

Because there are many combinations of genetic factors that result in a variety of 1-RM potentials and number of reps achieved with different percentages of a 1-RM, determining NA/CNS potential is not an exact science. However, it can be estimated in some cases, particularly when unusual results are produced by someone who does not "look the part." It is subjective, however estimating a person's NA/CNS potential can be done by:

1. Estimating their strength potential based on gender, body type in terms of height and weight, and body fat percentage. That will assign them a relative strength score (RSS) and classify them as either average, below average, or above average.

2. Sub-maximal resistances to MMF tests like the MU/fiber type tests.

ESTIMATING RELATIVE STRENGTH

Use the following male and female charts to estimate one's RSS (diagrams 10 and 11). Locate the height and weight range at the top of the respective chart, then locate the estimated body fat percentage on left. Where those bisect is the estimated RSS. Strength potential in this case defined by 1-RM ability in whatever exercises are used. Examples:

A male who is 5'-9" (175 cm.), 190 lbs. (86 kgs.), and 16% body fat would have an RSS of 6. This would be average (middle white area).

A male who is 6'-2" (188 cm.), 240 lbs. (109 kgs.), and 11% body fat would have an RSS of 9.5. This would be above average (green area).

A female who is 5'-5" (165 cm.), 148 lbs. (67 kgs.), and 26% body fat would have an RSS of 3.5. This would be below average (red area).

Other factors obviously affect strength output (skeletal leverage, MU/fiber type quantity and distribution, training status, etc.) but determining an RSS is the first step in estimating NA/CNS potential. It offers a "what they should be able to do" category prior to conducting specific submaximal resistances to MMF tests to better determine ability. If their body type suggests they should be able to display great strength – but exhibit below average ability – it could be due to a below average NA/CNS potential. Conversely, if their body type says below average strength ability – but they display an inordinate amount of force output – that points to a possible above average NA/CNS potential they were born with. Again, it's subjective but it may explain those abnormal abilities some people possess.

MALES																					
HEIGHT (ft./in.)	5'-2" - 5'-4"		5'-5" - 5'-8"				5'-9" - 6'-0"					6'-1" - 6'-4"					6'-5" +				
WEIGHT (lbs.)	115-135	136-155	140-159	160-179	180-199	200-219	145-164	165-184	185-204	205-224	225-244	160-179	180-199	200-219	220-239	240-259	190-209	210-229	230-249	250-269	270 +
HEIGHT (cm.)	157 - 162		165 - 173				175 - 183					185 - 193					196 +				
WEIGHT (kgs.)	52-61	62-70	64-72	73-81	82-90	91-100	66-75	75-84	84-93	93-102	102-111	73-81	82-90	91-100	100-109	109-118	86-95	95-104	105-113	114-122	123 +
% BODY FAT	RELATIVE STRENGTH SCORE																				
< 5%	9.5	10	9	9.5	10	10.5	9	9.5	10	10.5	11	9.5	10	10.5	11	11.5	10	10.5	11	11.5	12
6 - 8%	8.5	9	8	8.5	9	9.5	8	8.5	9	9.5	10	8.5	9	9.5	10	10.5	9	9.5	10	10.5	11
9 - 11%	7.5	8	7	7.5	8	8.5	7	7.5	8	8.5	9	7.5	8	8.5	9	9.5	8	8.5	9	9.5	10
12 - 14%	6.5	7	6	6.5	7	7.5	6	6.5	7	7.5	8	6.5	7	7.5	8	8.5	7	7.5	8	8.5	9
15 - 17%	5.5	6	5	5.5	6	6.5	5	5.5	6	6.5	7	5.5	6	6.5	7	7.5	6	6.5	7	7.5	8
18 - 20%	4.5	5	4	4.5	5	5.5	4	4.5	5	5.5	6	4.5	5	5.5	6	6.5	5	5.5	6	6.5	7
21 - 23%	3.5	4	3	3.5	4	4.5	3	3.5	4	4.5	5	3.5	4	4.5	5	5.5	4	4.5	5	5.5	6
24 - 26%	2.5	3	2	2.5	3	3.5	2	2.5	3	3.5	4	2.5	3	3.5	4	4.5	3	3.5	4	4.5	5
27 - 29%	1.5	2	1	1.5	2	2.5	1	1.5	2	2.5	3	1.5	2	2.5	3	3.5	2	2.5	3	3.5	4
30 - 32%	0.5	1	0	0.5	1	1.5	0	0.5	1	1.5	2	0.5	1	1.5	2	2.5	1	1.5	2	2.5	3
33 - 35%	-0.5	0	-1	-0.5	0	0.5	-1	-0.5	0	0.5	1	-0.5	0	0.5	1	1.5	0	0.5	1	1.5	2
> 36%	-1.5	-1	-2	-1.5	-1	-0.5	-2	-1.5	-1	-0.5	0	-1.5	-1	-0.5	0	0.5	-1	-0.5	0	0.5	1

Above Average Strength Potential =	12 to 8.5
Average Strength Potential =	8 to 4.5
Below Average Strength Potential =	4 >

Diagram 10: Male Relative Strength Score

FEMALES																
HEIGHT (ft./in.)	4'-10" - 5'-1"		5'-2" - 5'-5"				5'-6" - 5'-9"				5'-10" - 6'-1"			6'-2" +		
WEIGHT (lbs.)	80-100	101-120	110-130	131-150	151-170	171-190	125-145	146-165	166-185	186-205	140-160	161-180	181-200	161-180	181-200	201 +
HEIGHT (cm.)	147 - 155		157 - 165				168 - 175				178 - 185			188 +		
WEIGHT (kgs.)	36-45	46-55	50-59	60-68	69-77	78-86	57-66	66-75	75-84	85-93	64-73	73-82	82-91	73-82	82-91	92 +
% BODY FAT	RELATIVE STRENGTH SCORE															
< 10%	9.5	10	9	9.5	10	10.5	9.5	10	10.5	11	10.5	11	11.5	11	11.5	12
11 - 13%	8.5	9	8	8.5	9	9.5	8.5	9	9.5	10	9.5	10	10.5	10	10.5	11
14 - 16%	7.5	8	7	7.5	8	8.5	7.5	8	8.5	9	8.5	9	9.5	9	9.5	10
17 - 19%	6.5	7	6	6.5	7	7.5	6.5	7	7.5	8	7.5	8	8.5	8	8.5	9
20 - 22%	5.5	6	5	5.5	6	6.5	5.5	6	6.5	7	6.5	7	7.5	7	7.5	8
23 - 25%	4.5	5	4	4.5	5	5.5	4.5	5	5.5	6	5.5	6	6.5	6	6.5	7
26 - 28%	3.5	4	3	3.5	4	4.5	3.5	4	4.5	5	4.5	5	5.5	5	5.5	6
29 - 31%	2.5	3	2	2.5	3	3.5	2.5	3	3.5	4	3.5	4	4.5	4	4.5	5
32 - 34%	1.5	2	1	1.5	2	2.5	1.5	2	2.5	3	2.5	3	3.5	3	3.5	4
35 - 37%	0.5	1	0	0.5	1	1.5	0.5	1	1.5	2	1.5	2	2.5	2	2.5	3
38 - 40%	-0.5	0	-1	-0.5	0	0.5	-0.5	-1	0.5	1	0.5	1	1.5	1	1.5	2
> 41%	-1.5	-1	-2	-1.5	-1	-0.5	-1.5	-1	-0.5	0	-0.5	0	0.5	0	0.5	1

Above Average Strength Potential =	12 to 8.5
Average Strength Potential =	8 to 4.5
Below Average Strength Potential =	4 >

Diagram 11: Female Relative Strength Score

SUBMAXIMAL RESISTANCE TESTS

To estimate NA/CNS potential, three separate MMF tests with different percentages of a 1-RM can be used: 70%, 80%, and 90%. They are noted in diagram 12. It is best to do each test with complete recovery between them (i.e., on separate days when unfatigued as per the MU/fiber type tests). The number of max reps completed unassisted with each percentage resistance can help predict ability for the specific exercise performed.

Estimating Neurological Ability / Central Nervous System Potential

% of 1-RM Resistance	Reps to MMF	Estimated NA/CNS Potential
70%	9 to 12	Above Average
	15 to 20	Average
	25+	Below Average
80%	4 to 7	Above Average
	9 to 13	Average
	15+	Below Average
90%	1 or 2	Above Average
	3 to 6	Average
	7+	Below Average

Diagram 12: Estimating NA/CNS Potential Based on Reps to MMF With Various Percentages of a 1-RM

SUBJECT COMPARISONS

Subject 1 could have an *average strength* potential body:

- Male.
- 6'-1" 210 lbs. (185 cm./95 kgs.)
- 16% body fat.
- **RSS = 6.5**.

Standing barbell press 1-RM = 145 lbs./66 kgs.:

- 70% (102 lbs./46 kgs.) for **16 reps to MMF** = average NA/CNS potential.
- 80% (116 lbs./53 kgs.) for **10 reps to MMF** = average NA/CNS potential.
- 90% (131 lbs./59 kgs.) for **5 reps to MMF** = average NA/CNS potential.

Summary: Subject 1 looks the part and displays the part. He has an estimated average strength potential and is average strong in the standing barbell press. He possesses ability that shows average NA/CNS potential in that exercise due the ability to perform an average number of reps with submaximal resistances. His 1-RM strength reflects his local muscle endurance ability.

Alternative explanation: *below average NA/CNS potential* and a MU/ fiber type quantity and distribution of *average type 1, below average 2A,* and *above average 2X?*

☙ ❧

Subject 2 could have an *above average strength* potential body:

- Male.
- 5′-11″ 206 lbs. (180 cm./94 kgs.)
- 10% body fat.
- **RSS = 8.5**.

Standing barbell press 1-RM = 115 lbs./52 kgs.

- 70% (81 lbs./37 kgs.) for **24 reps to MMF** = below average NA/ CNS potential.
- 80% (92 lbs./42 kgs.) for **17 reps to MMF** = below average NA/ CNS potential.
- 90% (104 lbs./47 kgs.) for **8 reps to MMF** = below average NA/ CNS potential.

Summary: Subject 2 looks the part, but it is not manifested in his standing barbell press 1-RM ability of 115 lbs./52 kgs. He has an estimated above average strength potential but is sadly relatively weak. He possesses ability that shows below average NA/CNS potential in the standing barbell press due to the ability to perform an above average number of reps with lighter resistances but an inability to recruit many MUs/fibers in one maximum effort, hence the low 1-RM.

Alternative explanation: *average NA/CNS potential* and a MU/fiber type quantity and distribution of *above average type 1, average 2A,* and *below average 2X?*

☙ ❧

Subject 3 could have a *below average strength* potential body.

- Male.
- 5′-11″ 206 lbs. (180 cm./94 kgs.). Same height, weight, and gender as subject 1.
- 24% body fat (less muscle mass).
- **RSS = 3.5**.

Standing barbell press 1-RM = 180 lbs./82 kgs.

- 70% (126 lbs./57 kgs.) for **9 reps to MMF** = above average NA/CNS potential.

- 80% (144 lbs./65 kgs.) for **5 reps to MMF** = above average NA/CNS potential.

- 90% (162 lbs./74 kgs.) for **2 reps to MMF** = above average NA/CNS potential.

Summary: Subject 3 is the same height and weight as subject 1 but possesses below average strength potential due to being 24% fat and having less functional muscle mass in those pressing muscles. He should be weaker however he can hoist a significant amount of resistance in the standing barbell press. He possesses ability that depicts an above average NA/CNS potential because he's not able to perform many reps with submaximal resistances. He is exceptionally strong in that he can recruit many MUs/fibers in a single maximum effort but because of that he uses more each rep with lighter resistances. That leaves him with a lower reserve pool to recruit from (less local muscle endurance).

Alternative explanation: *average NA/CNS potential* and a MU/fiber type quantity and distribution of *average type 1, way below average 2A,* and *way above average 2X?*

※ ※

Subject 4 could have an *average strength potential* body.

- Female.

- 5'-5" 156 lbs. (165 cm./71 kgs.).

- 23% body fat.

- **RSS = 5.**

Leg press 1-RM = 275 lbs./125 kgs. (on the specific leg press device).

- 70% (193 lbs./88 kgs.) for **21 reps to MMF** = below average NA/CNS potential.

- 80% (220 lbs./100 kgs.) for **15 reps to MMF** = below average NA/CNS potential.

- 90% (248 lbs./113 kgs.) for **7 reps to MMF** = below average NA/CNS potential.

Summary: Subject 4 is estimated to have average strength potential based on her relative strength score data. She has a 1-RM leg press of 275 lbs./125 kgs. on that specific leg press device (leverage and mechanics differ between manufacturers' designs). Assuming that amount would be considered average ability, she possesses average strength. She also possesses ability that depicts a below average NA/CNS potential due to her ability to perform a slight above average number of reps with submaximal resistances (combined average strength and slight above average local muscle endurance).

Alternative explanation: *above average NA/CNS potential* and a MU/ fiber type quantity and distribution of *above average type 1, average 2A,* and *below average 2X?*

☙ ❧

Subject 5 could have a *below average strength potential* body.

- Female.
- 5'-10" 140 lbs. (178 cm./64 kgs.).
- 30% body fat.
- **RSS = 3.5.**

Leg press 1-RM = 135 lbs./61 kgs. (on the specific leg press device).

- 70% (95 lbs./43 kgs.) for **16 reps to MMF** = average NA/CNS potential.
- 80% (108 lbs./49 kgs.) for **11 reps to MMF** = average NA/CNS potential.
- 90% (122 lbs./55 kgs.) for **4 reps to MMF** = average NA/CNS potential.

Summary : Subject 5 is estimated to have below average strength potential based on her relative strength score data. She is tall, seemingly thin, but under that skin is 30% body fat. Essentially, she does not possess a lot of muscle to generate a high level of force. Her 1-RM leg press of only 135 lbs./61 kgs. on the same leg press device as subject 4 reflects that. In fact, it is way below average. However, her ability with the percentages to MMF equate to an average NA/CNS potential, possibly due to her below average strength coupled with the usual MU/fiber reserve that goes with it, but not as much as normally would be evident with a below average NA/CNS potential. She is a relatively weak person but can exhibit at least average local muscle endurance.

Alternative explanation: *below average NA/CNS potential* and a MU/ fiber type quantity and distribution of *above average type 1, average 2A, and below average 2X?*

⧗ ⧗

Subject 6 could have an *average strength potential* body.

- Female.
- 5'-3" 165 lbs. (160 cm./75 kgs.).
- 19% body fat.
- **RSS = 7.**

Leg press 1-RM = 265 lbs./120 kgs. (on the specific leg press device).

- 70% (186 lbs./84 kgs.) for **10 reps to MMF** = above average NA/CNS potential.
- 80% (212 lbs./96 kgs.) for **6 reps to MMF** = above average NA/ CNS potential.
- 90% (239 lbs./108 kgs.) for **2 reps to MMF** = above average NA/CNS potential.

Summary: subject 6 has similar average strength like subject 4, but is shorter, slightly heavier, and leaner. She has more muscle to work with but does not exhibit significant strength. Even though her 1-RM is slightly below subject 4, her ability with the submaximal resistances is much less in comparison, indicating a possible above average NA/CNS potential. Fewer reps performed with submaximal resistances is normally the case with the above average NA/CNS potential, but it also usually means greater strength potential, which she does not possess. Therefore, the ability of subject 6 is more affected by her MU/fiber type quantity and distribution in the leg pressing muscles.

Alternative explanation: *below average NA/CNS potential* and a MU/ fiber type quantity and distribution of *average type 1, below average 2A, and above average 2X?*

THE FINAL WORD ON ESTIMATING STRENGTH POTENTIAL AND NA/CNS POTENTIAL

It is impossible to determine strength ability on physical appearance alone. One's amount of functional muscle mass may help speculate relative ability because — all other factors equal — more muscle mass =

more strength potential. That is a starting point, but more information is needed to make a more accurate estimate.

Most of the population has an average NA/CNS potential, and any differences in strength potential stem from the quantity and distribution of the three MU/fiber types in the working muscles. If there is an unusual ability displayed – either way above or way below average strength – it is likely due to an above or below average NA/CNS potential.

As a rule, estimating NA/CNS potential via maximum rep tests with various percentages of a 1-RM can be used. Those results can then be compared to one's 1-RM and body type to make a subjective evaluation of ability. On that, all other factors being equal:

An above average NA/CNS potential usually means...

1. A greater relative strength/higher 1-RM, but lesser relative local muscle endurance due to a smaller MU/fiber reserve pool.

2. One does not "look the part" but displays exceptional strength.

A below average NA/CNS potential usually means...

1. A lesser relative strength/lower 1-RM, but greater relative local muscle endurance due to a larger MU/fiber reserve pool.

2. One "looks the part" but displays poor strength.

INCREASING MUSCLE SIZE

There are essentially two ways of increasing limb and torso girth/size: by increasing fat storage or by increasing muscle mass. Obviously, becoming larger via fat storage is not the viable option because it's both unhealthy and unsightly. Muscle mass increase (hypertrophy) is more desirable but it will take a lot of work and discipline for most people. Again, it's the genetic factor that determines the optimal number of reps to perform relative to one's potential to grow muscle. The key factors are:

- Resistance training experience: trained vs. untrained.

- The current volume of muscle mass...small/thin, average, or large/thick.

- The quantity and distribution of the three MU/fiber types in the relevant muscles one is seeking to enlarge.

Rationale:

- Untrained people have a relative total muscle volume that has not been stimulated to grow.

- An average volume of muscle will have the greatest potential to grow muscle because 1) small/thin muscles have little potential and 2) large/thick muscles are already large. This leaves the between-size average person with the most potential, relatively speaking.

- Possessing more type 2X MUs/fibers – the largest of the three – allows for more growth potential provided they are stimulated to grow.

All other factors being equal, Diagram 13 lists in order the combination of factors that affect the ability to grow muscle from the *most potential* to the *least potential* (a score of 4.5 has the most potential and 1.25 has the least).

Independent of genetic endowment anyone can improve muscle size if they train using a progressive resistance program. If one has been training for years (and has already created muscle growth via proper progressive training), obviously they are limited in the amount of further growth that can occur. Conversely, if just beginning a program they are "untapped" and have more potential to grow muscle.

MU/Fiber Type Quantity	Status	Muscle Volume	Score
Above Average 2X - Average 2A - Below Average Type 1	Untrained	Average Muscle Mass	4.5
Average 2X - Above Average 2A - Below Average Type 1	Untrained	Average Muscle Mass	4.25
Above Average 2X - Below Average 2A - Average Type 1	Untrained	Average Muscle Mass	4
Above Average 2X - Average 2A - Below Average Type 1	Untrained	Small/Thin Muscle	4
Below Average 2X - Above Average 2A - Average Type 1	Untrained	Average Muscle Mass	3.75
Average 2X - Above Average 2A - Below Average Type 1	Untrained	Small/Thin Muscle	3.75
Average 2X - Below Average 2A - Above Average Type 1	Untrained	Average Muscle Mass	3.5
Above Average 2X - Below Average 2A - Average Type 1	Untrained	Small/Thin Muscle	3.5
Above Average 2X - Average 2A - Below Average Type 1	Untrained	Large/Thick Muscle	3.5
Above Average 2X - Average 2A - Below Average Type 1	Trained	Average Muscle Mass	3.5
Below Average 2X - Average 2A - Above Average Type 1	Untrained	Average Muscle Mass	3.25
Below Average 2X - Above Average 2A - Average Type 1	Untrained	Small/Thin Muscle	3.25
Average 2X - Above Average 2A - Below Average Type 1	Untrained	Large/Thick Muscle	3.25
Average 2X - Above Average 2A - Below Average Type 1	Trained	Average Muscle Mass	3.25
Average 2X - Below Average 2A - Above Average Type 1	Untrained	Small/Thin Muscle	3
Above Average 2X - Below Average 2A - Average Type 1	Untrained	Large/Thick Muscle	3
Above Average 2X - Below Average 2A - Average Type 1	Trained	Average Muscle Mass	3
Above Average 2X - Average 2A - Below Average Type 1	Trained	Small/Thin Muscle	3
Below Average 2X - Average 2A - Above Average Type 1	Untrained	Small/Thin Muscle	2.75
Below Average 2X - Above Average 2A - Average Type 1	Untrained	Large/Thick Muscle	2.75
Below Average 2X - Above Average 2A - Average Type 1	Trained	Average Muscle Mass	2.75
Average 2X - Above Average 2A - Below Average Type 1	Trained	Small/Thin Muscle	2.75
Average 2X - Below Average 2A - Above Average Type 1	Untrained	Large/Thick Muscle	2.5
Average 2X - Below Average 2A - Above Average Type 1	Trained	Average Muscle Mass	2.5
Above Average 2X - Below Average 2A - Average Type 1	Trained	Small/Thin Muscle	2.5
Above Average 2X - Average 2A - Below Average Type 1	Trained	Large/Thick Muscle	2.5
Below Average 2X - Average 2A - Above Average Type 1	Untrained	Large/Thick Muscle	2.25
Below Average 2X - Average 2A - Above Average Type 1	Trained	Average Muscle Mass	2.25
Below Average 2X - Above Average 2A - Average Type 1	Trained	Small/Thin Muscle	2.25
Average 2X - Above Average 2A - Below Average Type 1	Trained	Large/Thick Muscle	2.25
Average 2X - Below Average 2A - Above Average Type 1	Trained	Small/Thin Muscle	2
Above Average 2X - Below Average 2A - Average Type 1	Trained	Large/Thick Muscle	2
Below Average 2X - Average 2A - Above Average Type 1	Trained	Small/Thin Muscle	1.75
Below Average 2X - Above Average 2A - Average Type 1	Trained	Large/Thick Muscle	1.75
Average 2X - Below Average 2A - Above Average Type 1	Trained	Large/Thick Muscle	1.5
Below Average 2X - Average 2A - Above Average Type 1	Trained	Large/Thick Muscle	1.25

Diagram 13: Potential to Grow Muscle Based on MU/Fiber Type Quantity, Training Status, and Current Muscle Volume.

PUTTING IT ALL TOGETHER – THE OPTIMAL NUMBER OF REPS TO PERFORM FOR INCREASING STRENGTH, POWER, LOCAL MUSCLE ENDURANCE, AND MUSCLE SIZE

For the genetically average person performing any type of progressive resistance training program that contains a combination of high, moderate, and low reps will enhance overall force output ability. This applies to the expressions of strength (maximum force in one effort), power (quick application of that max force), and local muscle endurance (sustained force output over time/multiple bouts). It also applies to hypertrophy (muscle growth) in as much as any MU/fiber that is recruited and fatigued can grow larger relative to its potential: 2X having the greatest potential to increase in size, then type 2A, and type 1 having the least.

Others may require slight variations and/or more emphasis on a specific number of reps if their genetic makeup is above or below average due in part to their NA/CNS potential. Keep in mind the previous 10-RM and 35-RM comparison examples of possible outcomes between subjects with above and below average NA/CNS potentials combined with various quantities and distributions of the three MU/fiber types. Compared to an average NA/CNS potential, their abilities will differ even more, which would require more experimentation to determine more accurate reps to prescribe.

Prescribing an optimal number of reps for everyone is prudent, but it should also be done for the different muscle groups each possesses. That is, one may need higher reps around 20 to train the lower body (squat, dead lift, and leg press), around 12 for the back torso (seated rows/pulldowns), and possibly eight for the front torso (decline, flat, incline, and overhead presses). So, using the max rep tests to MMF with percentages of a 1-RM may help determine more productive target reps for individual exercises each person will perform.

The following diagram can be used when prescribing optimal reps in resistance training program design. The recommended reps are actually rep ranges which better account for variations in abilities among the population relative to all genetic differences (i.e., 6 to 10, 12 to 16, 20 to 25). Understand these points as well:

- Proper stimulation of muscle is a result of time-under-tension and not simply completing "x" number of reps. Because the traditional means of programming reps is usually done by assigning rep numbers and not elapsed clock time, rep ranges do represent a certain time-under-tension.

- Rep ranges better facilitate simple progression. Knowing progressive training entails increasing the amount of resistance and/or performing more reps over a sequence of training sessions, rep ranges 1) allow for slow but sure progression and 2) account for sub-par training days.

Essentially, rep ranges allow for gradual progression via an extra rep (or even a half-rep) each forthcoming session with the same resistance, then a resistance increase at the appropriate time. They are not solely about constant resistance increases each session that would quickly halt progress. They allow for those sub-par days when one may not show improvement from the previous session (which is normal for all trainees).

Years of training experience, the performance of 1-RM percentages to MMF tests, and a bit of common sense can all be used to determine sensible rep ranges for optimal development pursuant to one's goal(s). The data in diagram 14 can be used as a guide for that. It offers rep prescription options based on all combinations of MU/fiber type quantities and distributions in conjunction with average, above average, and below average NA/CNS potentials.

OPTIMAL NUMBER OF REPS TO PERFORM
Based on NA/CNS Potential & MU/Fiber Type Quantity & Distribution

Key:
MUs/fibers: 1 = Type 1   2A = Type 2A   2X = Type 2X
Quantity: A = Average   AA = Above Average   BA = Below Average
Potential: WBA = Way below average   BA = Below average   SBA = Slight below average   A = Average   SAA = Slight above average   AA = Above average   WAA

RECOMMENDED REP RANGES OR % OF A 1-RM TO USE

NA/CNS POTENTIAL:			AVERAGE			ABOVE AVERAGE			BELOW AVERAGE		
REP CATEGORY:			LOW	MODERATE	HIGH	LOW	MODERATE	HIGH	LOW	MODERATE	HIGH
MU/Fiber Type Quantity 1 2A 2X	Strength Potential	Endurance Potential	Rep Range / % 1-RM	Rep Range / % 1-RM	Rep Range / % 1-RM	Rep Range / % 1-RM	Rep Range / % 1-RM	Rep Range / % 1-RM	Rep Range / % 1-RM	Rep Range / % 1-RM	Rep Range / % 1-RM
AA A BA	WBA	AA	7 - 10 / 82.5%	13 - 17 / 72.5%	21 - 26 / 62.5%	6 - 8 / 77.5%	11 - 14 / 67.5%	19 - 24 / 57.5%	8 - 11 / 87.5%	15 - 20 / 77.5%	23 - 28 / 67.5%
AA BA A	BA	SBA	6 - 9 / 85%	11 - 14 / 75%	19 - 24 / 65%	5 - 7 / 80%	9 - 12 / 70%	17 - 22 / 60%	7 - 10 / 90%	13 - 17 / 80%	21 - 26 / 70%
A AA BA	SBA	WAA	4 - 7 / 87.5%	9 - 12 / 77.5%	17 - 22 / 67.5%	4 - 5 / 82.5%	8 - 11 / 72.5%	15 - 20 / 62.5%	6 - 8 / 92.5%	11 - 14 / 82.5%	19 - 24 / 72.5%
Each @ Average	A	A	3 - 6 / 90%	8 - 11 / 80%	15 - 20 / 70%	3 - 4 / 85%	7 - 10 / 75%	13 - 17 / 65%	5 - 7 / 95%	9 - 12 / 85%	17 - 22 / 75%
A BA AA	SAA	WBA	2 - 4 / 92.5%	7 - 10 / 82.5%	13 - 17 / 72.5%	2 - 3 / 87.5%	6 - 8 / 77.5%	11 - 14 / 67.5%	4 - 6 / 96.5%	8 - 11 / 86.5%	15 - 20 / 76.5%
BA AA A	AA	SAA	1 - 3 / 95%	6 - 9 / 85%	11 - 14 / 75%	1 - 2 / 90%	5 - 7 / 80%	9 - 12 / 70%	3 - 5 / 98%	7 - 10 / 88%	13 - 17 / 78%
BA A AA	WAA	BA	1 - 2 / 97.5%	4 - 7 / 87.5%	9 - 12 / 77.5%	1 - 2 / 92.5%	4 - 5 / 82.5%	8 - 11 / 72.5%	2 - 4 / 99.5%	6 - 8 / 89.5%	12 - 15 / 79.5%

Diagram 14: Optimal Number of Reps to Perform Based on NA/CNS Potential and MU/Fiber Quantity and Distribution

WHICH ONE IS MORE IMPORTANT, THE NUMBER OF REPS PERFORMED (I.E., 15) OR AMOUNT OF TIME IT TAKES TO COMPLETE A SET (I.E., :45)?

Again, it is all about time under tension.

The energy systems function on time and intensity, not an arbitrary number of repetitions. How one performs the exercise regarding rep velocity and cadence dictates the energy system(s) involvement. One could perform 10 reps to muscle fatigue at an average velocity and cadence of :03 per rep for a total set time of :30 (:015 concentric/raising + :015 eccentric/lowering). This same person could perform 10 reps to muscle fatigue using a :05 per second rep velocity and cadence for a total set time of :50 (:025 per concentric/eccentric).

The amount of resistance used for both the :30 and :50 sets would need to be different due to the additional :20 it would take to reach muscle fatigue in the :50 set. Therefore, the entire resistance-recruitment-fatigue-time under tension scheme is different for each scenario. Essentially, the :50 set would be a lighter, higher rep set and the :30 set a heavier, lower rep set, both with the goal of achieving MMF. The set results would be dictated by their inherent MU/fiber type quantity and distribution and NA/CNS potential.

Because most trainees do not time their sets (unless they are using a purposely slow velocity and cadence overload protocol), a target rep goal number or range of reps is the standard means of performing sets and documenting progression. Provided all reps are completed consistently with the same velocity and cadence, using a specific range of reps (or specific target rep number) is easier to document. Regardless of how logged, assure to note the amount of resistance used and the number of reps completed for accurate progression. If using a timed overload protocol such as in deliberate slow training, be sure to record the time under tension as the marker for accurate progression.

SHOULD MULTIPLE SETS (I.E., TWO+) BE PERFORMED FOR BEST RESULTS?

The optimal number of sets to perform topic often-times elicits emotional responses from various factions in the resistance training world. Arguing for one way or the other by covering all relevant factors in detail using thousands of words and hundreds of minutes is beyond the scope of this book. What follows is an overview of both options –

either one set only or multiple sets - regarding the pragmatic use of either one. One can then decide which is more prudent when concocting a relevant resistance training program.

> NOTE: The one set vs. multiple sets debate has raged on for years. Many studies have been conducted that compared results from a one set/exercise against multiple sets/exercise. The outcomes are mixed but both methods improve muscle force outputs.

One factor to consider is the goal of the workout session. Is the session dedicated solely to addressing all major muscle structures to efficiently recruit and fatigue the greatest quantity of MUs/fibers, so they grow and become stronger? That can be accomplished with a minimal number of total sets performed that use the immediate ATP stores, quick ATP replenishment via the CK reaction, and then glycolysis to produce energy if the reps go beyond 15 to 20. If the goal is to seek a conditioning effect by stressing the cardio-respiratory system using multiple exercise bouts, higher rep sets, and/or minimal recovery time between bouts, that can be accomplished with a bit more workout volume, a la circuit-type resistance training.

Either way, many options will work provided one's goals are reached. Whether it is 15 minutes or one hour, exuding 100% effort to each set/exercise bout is still the bottom line. Think train hard and train brief. Brief in terms of a reasonable number of total workouts sets each session, eschewing unnecessary and meaningless work. If you're not convinced, read on...

Doing something is 100% greater than doing nothing.

Doing something is better than doing nothing. Doing something is 100% better than doing nothing. Performing one set is 100% better than not performing one set. If a person gives 100% all-out effort on one set it is 100% better than not going all out. If that person performs one all-out set of eight exercises that address the entire body, it is 100% better than not doing those exercises. If that person gives 100% on those eight exercises twice per week, on non-consecutive days (i.e., Tuesday and Friday), and for 10 weeks total, that commitment is 100% better than not training hard, briefly, and infrequently for those 10 weeks. Will that person who committed to that 10-week program be stronger, more powerful, possess more muscle mass, and better able to express better local muscle endurance compared to a person who committed absolutely zero time to training? 100% yes. Think about that when your excuse is "I just don't have the time to train." It is 100% false.

In that context, using one set per exercise works 100% of the time.

Time efficiency.

Unless you work at a gym or have a means to train at home, you will need to schedule time for transit to the facility. You'll also need to time change into workout clothing, warm up, train, cool down, tend to post-workout personal hygiene, and again do the travel thing back to work or your abode. Remember, having little time is no excuse not to train, but at least some time does need to be scheduled into your weekly routine. You know where I am going with this if you heeded the rationale behind the previous 100%-greater-than-zero discussion.

Result-producing resistance training is hard. And it should be. If, however, one truly does work hard in each set performed, only a minimal number of sets are needed. It comes down to this: once an overload stress is placed upon a muscle or group of muscles the mission is accomplished. That's it. No more stimulus is required. Time to move on.

Hard, brief, and minimal-volume-of-sets training is schedule-friendly, especially when the entire travel to, pre-prep, post-prep, and travel back factors are included. Do you only have 45 minutes to commit twice per week? That can work. How about three days but only 30 minutes each day? No problem. And don't become a member of the typical "I-go-to-the-gym-five-days-per-week" crowd. Most of that ilk 1) do not train hard, 2) perform a high volume of unstimulating sets, 3) stay for two+ hours and spends half of that time fiddling with their music player and ear buds, 4) may train hard but over-train due to lack of necessary recovery days, and/or 5) need to spend many hours per week in the gym to fulfill a social need or quell an insecurity issue.

One set per muscle group, one set per exercise, or mini-multiple sets per muscle group or exercise?

Time-efficient workouts can be constructed many ways. A program that includes 10 different exercises at one set for each muscle group will work. A program that includes 12 total exercises but two sets per muscle group will work. A program that includes five different exercises for three sets of each – a total workout volume of 15 sets - will work.

The key element is the effort expended each set. As noted, working hard each set should be the goal. If so, a minimal number of sets is only required. A multitude of research has been conducted on the comparison between one vs. multiple sets. They both produce results.

On that, because there is no magic number of sets that is optimal, it is one's prerogative if they desire more volume. This is acceptable if engaging in circuit resistance training where a cardio-respiratory demand is desired. It's also acceptable to perform one to three different exercises for a specific body part (i.e., leg day only). That is still time efficient as opposed to some high-volume programs that assign five+ sets each for three to four exercises for a single muscle group. That is unnecessary.

Most H.I.T. and time-efficient protocols prescribe a single set per exercise, but it may be from one to three per muscle group. It could be something like these:

Glutes and quads: one set each of a plate-load leg press, machine squat, and dumbbell dead lift.

Pectorals: one set each of an incline press, body-weight dip, and machine chest press.

Remember, a lot of things work provided they are reasonable.

Circling back to the proven point that doing something is 100% better than doing absolutely nothing, the following format would work if it was performed with 100% effort on a consistent basis (i.e., two or three days per week on non-consecutive days):

- Pulldown or chin up x 1 set of 10–14 reps (or max reps if doing the chin up).
- Dumbbell squat x 1 set of 20-25 reps.
- Decline press or dip x 1 set of 8-12 reps (or max reps if doing the dip).
- Leg curl x 1 set of 10-14 reps.
- Bent-over row x 1 set of 8-12 reps.
- Dumbbell side lateral raise x 1 set of 10-14 reps.
- Bicycle crunch x 1 set of max reps.

Seven exercises, one set each, 100% all-out effort, and performed on a regular basis = guaranteed results when compared to doing absolutely nothing.

The key take-away is some volume for a specific muscle group is reasonable. Just make sure the total session volume is not excessive.

WHY DOES INCREASING MUSCLE STRENGTH INCREASE LOCAL MUSCLE ENDURANCE?

As discussed previously, one who trains progressively to improve muscle force capacity will develop a greater reserve pool of MUs/fibers as compared to their initial non-trained status. In extended sets performed to MMF, possessing greater strength means fewer MUs/fibers are recruited in the initial reps which leaves more available to extend rep performance as fatigue accumulates.

Examples:

Day 1 ability:

> 1-RM = 200 lbs./91 kgs.
>
> 10-RM = 150 lbs./68 kgs.

Day 60 ability:

> 1-RM now 230 lbs./105 kgs.
>
> New 10-RM = 172.5 lbs./78 kgs.
>
> The initial 10-RM resistance of 150 lbs./68 kgs can now be completed for 15 reps.

WHAT ARE THE OPTIMAL NUMBER OF REPS TO PERFORM WHEN RESISTANCE TRAINING FOR FAT LOSS?

Thank you for understanding the need for resistance training in an effective fat loss program!

Resistance training programs that facilitate fat loss can be designed many ways. The most important point to remember is whatever work is done in the weight room will not be as effective for fat loss compared to proper food intake. 80% of the fat loss work involves the dietary component, not how may reps to perform in a dumbbell squat.

Before discussing the optimal number of reps for fat loss, please heed this useful information.

Most fat loss programs should include a calorie deficit. That is, fewer calories consumed than expended. Provided other factors are accounted for, this promotes the loss of adipose fat stores (the pinchable stuff). In the calorie-deficit mode the goal should be to consume a reasonable diet without becoming exasperated by time-consuming calorie counting, expensive trips to the supermarket, or purchasing even more expensive supplements. Consume adequate proteins, good fats, and vitamin and mineral-rich vegetables and fruit (unless one is on the Keto Diet). A concerted effort should be made to avoid processed food (bad carbs) and other chemicals that continually spike insulin levels that promote fat storage. And it is okay to have a cheat day here or there. It is not glum and doom if one cannot completely eschew their favorite cheat items. Think about this: if seven out of every 10 meals consumed are healthy, that is pretty darn good. It offers a little wiggle room to stray occasionally in this world chock-full of so many sub-par food temptations encountered everywhere.

One potential problem with the fewer calories going in is for one's metabolism will slow to conserve energy and maintain one's status quo. So, one needs to give the body a reason to keep using calories, especially post-workout. The way to do that is create a high demand on the muscles via resistance training. If done, the body must use that stored adipose fat as energy to recover and refuel during the energy-replenishing and muscle-rebuilding recovery downtime.

And know that muscle gives one better "shape" compared to fat. Muscle is more functional than fat. Muscle is sexier than fat. Male or female, it is all about resistance training with intensity and addressing all major muscle groups in some reasonable manner.

An excessive amount of low-level work like distance running, slogging away on a treadmill for an hour, a few miles of brisk walking, or a pathetic 30:00 yoga class are not great options for that. In fact, those types of exercise decrease muscle mass which further lowers metabolism and essentially promotes fat storage.

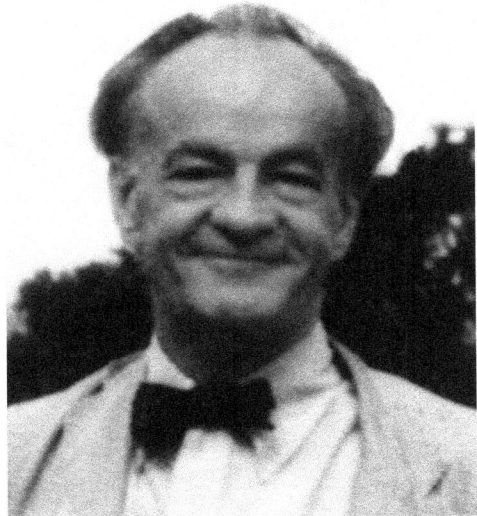

Figure 16 – Elwood Henneman (22)
The Father of Henneman's Size Principle of Motor Unit Recruitment

Now to that "How many reps to perform" question. There is no magic number of reps for fat loss. It's just about progressive training. One can use low to moderate reps. One can use moderate to high reps. Much depends on the optimal number of reps for each muscle group based on one's MU/fiber type quantity and distribution and NA/CNS potential. Regardless, it's all about getting to the gym and performing some type of resistance training to create overload on all major muscle structures to build or at least maintain muscle mass in the wake of fat loss calorie restriction.

APPENDICES

The following diagrams and figures were used to calculate and/or estimate MU/Fiber and Central Nervous System characteristics to determine hypothetical force output potentials of subjects regarding:

- Strength and local muscle endurance.

- NA/CNS abilities of either average, below average, or above average.

- MU/Fiber Units of Force recruitment and fatigue during 1-RM, 10-RM, and 35-RM events.

AVERAGE NA/CNS (70%) 700/1000						
MU/FIBER TYPE QUANTITY			STRENGTH POTENTIAL	ENDURANCE POTENTIAL	TOTAL POINTS	
					STR.	END.
1	2A	2X			(2A + 2X)	(1 + 2A)
ABOVE	AVERAGE	BELOW	WAY BELOW	ABOVE	4.5	7
ABOVE	BELOW	AVERAGE	BELOW	SLIGHT BELOW	5	5.5
AVERAGE	ABOVE	BELOW	SLIGHT BELOW	WAY ABOVE	5.5	7.5
AVERAGE	AVERAGE	AVERAGE	AVERAGE	AVERAGE	6	6
AVERAGE	BELOW	ABOVE	SLIGHT ABOVE	WAY BELOW	6.5	4.5
BELOW	ABOVE	AVERAGE	ABOVE	SLIGHT ABOVE	7	6.5
BELOW	AVERAGE	ABOVE	WAY ABOVE	BELOW	7.5	5

ABOVE AVERAGE NA/CNS (74%) 740/1000						
MU/FIBER TYPE QUANTITY			STRENGTH POTENTIAL	ENDURANCE POTENTIAL	TOTAL POINTS	
					STR.	END.
1	2A	2X			(2A – 2X)	(1 + 2A)
ABOVE	AVERAGE	BELOW	WAY BELOW	ABOVE	5.5	6
ABOVE	BELOW	AVERAGE	BELOW	SLIGHT BELOW	6	4.5
AVERAGE	ABOVE	BELOW	SLIGHT BELOW	WAY ABOVE	6.5	6.5
AVERAGE	AVERAGE	AVERAGE	AVERAGE	AVERAGE	7	5
AVERAGE	BELOW	ABOVE	SLIGHT ABOVE	WAY BELOW	7.5	3.5
BELOW	ABOVE	AVERAGE	ABOVE	SLIGHT ABOVE	8	5.5
BELOW	AVERAGE	ABOVE	WAY ABOVE	BELOW	8.5	4

BELOW AVERAGE NA/CNS (66%) 660/1000

MU/FIBER TYPE QUANTITY			STRENGTH POTENTIAL	ENDURANCE POTENTIAL	TOTAL POINTS	
					STR.	END.
1	2A	2X			(2A + 2X)	(1 + 2A)
ABOVE	AVERAGE	BELOW	WAY BELOW	ABOVE	3.5	8
ABOVE	BELOW	AVERAGE	BELOW	SLIGHT BELOW	4	6.5
AVERAGE	ABOVE	BELOW	SLIGHT BELOW	WAY ABOVE	4.5	8.5
AVERAGE	AVERAGE	AVERAGE	AVERAGE	AVERAGE	5	7
AVERAGE	BELOW	ABOVE	SLIGHT ABOVE	WAY BELOW	5.5	5.5
BELOW	ABOVE	AVERAGE	ABOVE	SLIGHT ABOVE	6	7.5
BELOW	AVERAGE	ABOVE	WAY ABOVE	BELOW	6.5	6

AVERAGE NA/CNS POTENTIAL (70%)

MU/FIBER TYPE ENDURANCE POINT VALUE BASED ON QUANTITY				MU/FIBER TYPE STRENGTH POINT VALUE BASED ON QUANTITY			
	1	2A	2X		1	2A	2X
BELOW AVERAGE	1.5	2	2.5	BELOW AVERAGE	1.5	1.5	2
AVERAGE	2.5	3.5	1.5	AVERAGE	2.5	2.5	3.5
ABOVE AVERAGE	3.5	5	0.5	ABOVE AVERAGE	3.5	3.5	5

ESTIMATED 1-RM RESISTANCE FROM COMBINED STRENGTH POINTS (2A + 2X) AND ESTIMATED 10-RM RESISTANCE USED FROM COMBINED ENDURANCE POINTS (1 + 2A)

10-RM

STRENGTH POINTS	STRENGTH CATEGORY	1-RM (lbs./kgs.)		ENDURANCE POINTS	ENDURANCE CATEGORY	% used for 10-RM	10-RM (lbs./kgs.)
4.5	WAY BELOW	266/121		7.5	WAY ABOVE	87.5%	233/106
5	BELOW	294/134		7	ABOVE	85%	250/114
5.5	SLIGHT BELOW	322/146		6.5	SLIGHT ABOVE	82.5%	266/121
6	AVERAGE	350/159		6	AVERAGE	80%	280/127
6.5	SLIGHT ABOVE	378/172		5.5	SLIGHT BELOW	77.5%	293/133
7	ABOVE	406/185		5	BELOW	75%	305/138
7.5	WAY ABOVE	434/197		4.5	WAY BELOW	72.5%	315/143

ABOVE AVERAGE NA/CNS POTENTIAL (74%)

MU/FIBER TYPE ENDURANCE POINT VALUE BASED ON QUANTITY				MU/FIBER TYPE STRENGTH POINT VALUE BASED ON QUANTITY			
	1	2A	2X		1	2A	2X
BELOW AVERAGE	1	1.5	2	BELOW AVERAGE	3	2	2.5
AVERAGE	2	3	1	AVERAGE	2	3	4
ABOVE AVERAGE	3	4.5	0	ABOVE AVERAGE	1	4	5.5

ESTIMATED 1-RM RESISTANCE FROM COMBINED STRENGTH POINTS (2A + 2X) AND ESTIMATED 10-RM RESISTANCE USED FROM COMBINED ENDURANCE POINTS (1 + 2A)

10-RM

STRENGTH POINTS	STRENGTH CATEGORY	1-RM (lbs./kgs.)		ENDURANCE POINTS	ENDURANCE CATEGORY	% used for 10-RM	10-RM (lbs./kgs.)
5.5	WAY BELOW	304/138		6.5	WAY ABOVE	82.5%	251/114
6	BELOW	336/153		6	ABOVE	80%	269/122
6.5	SLIGHT BELOW	368/167		5.5	SLIGHT ABOVE	77.5%	285/130
7	AVERAGE	400/182		5	AVERAGE	75%	300/136
7.5	SLIGHT ABOVE	432/196		4.5	SLIGHT BELOW	72.5%	313/142
8	ABOVE	464/211		4	BELOW	70%	325/148
8.5	WAY ABOVE	496/225		3.5	WAY BELOW	67.5%	335/152

BELOW AVERAGE NA/CNS POTENTIAL (66%)

MU/FIBER TYPE ENDURANCE POINT VALUE BASED ON QUANTITY				MU/FIBER TYPE STRENGTH POINT VALUE BASED ON QUANTITY			
	1	2A	2X		1	2A	2X
BELOW AVERAGE	2	2.5	3	BELOW AVERAGE	2	1	1.5
AVERAGE	3	4	2	AVERAGE	1	2	3
ABOVE AVERAGE	4	5.5	1	ABOVE AVERAGE	0	3	4.5

ESTIMATED 1-RM RESISTANCE FROM COMBINED STRENGTH POINTS (2A + 2X) AND ESTIMATED 10-RM RESISTANCE USED FROM COMBINED ENDURANCE POINTS (1 + 2A)

10-RM

STRENGTH POINTS	STRENGTH CATEGORY	1-RM (lbs./kgs.)		ENDURANCE POINTS	ENDURANCE CATEGORY	% used for 10-RM	10-RM (lbs./kgs.)
3.5	WAY BELOW	228/104		8.5	WAY ABOVE	92.5%	211/96
4	BELOW	252/115		8	ABOVE	90%	227/103
4.5	SLIGHT BELOW	276/125		7.5	SLIGHT ABOVE	87.5%	242/110
5	AVERAGE	300/136		7	AVERAGE	85%	255/116
5.5	SLIGHT ABOVE	324/147		6.5	SLIGHT BELOW	82.5%	267/122
6	ABOVE	348/158		6	BELOW	80%	278/127
6.5	WAY ABOVE	372/169		5.5	WAY BELOW	77.5%	288/131

AVERAGE NA/CNS POTENTIAL (70%)

MU/FIBER TYPE ENDURANCE POINT VALUE BASED ON QUANTITY				MU/FIBER TYPE STRENGTH POINT VALUE BASED ON QUANTITY		
	1	2A	2X		1	2A	2X
BELOW AVERAGE	1.5	2	2.5	BELOW AVERAGE	2.5	1.5	2
AVERAGE	2.5	3.5	1.5	AVERAGE	1.5	2.5	3.5
ABOVE AVERAGE	3.5	5	0.5	ABOVE AVERAGE	0.5	3.5	5

ESTIMATED 1-RM RESISTANCE FROM COMBINED STRENGTH POINTS (2A + 2X) AND ESTIMATED 35-RM RESISTANCE USED FROM COMBINED ENDURANCE POINTS (1 + 2A)

35-RM

STRENGTH POINTS	STRENGTH CATEGORY	1-RM (lbs./kgs.)		ENDURANCE POINTS	ENDURANCE CATEGORY	% used for 35-RM	35-RM (lbs./kgs.)
4.5	WAY BELOW	209/95		7.5	WAY ABOVE	64%	134/61
5	BELOW	231/105		7	ABOVE	61%	141/64
5.5	SLIGHT BELOW	253/115		6.5	SLIGHT ABOVE	58%	147/67
6	AVERAGE	275/125		6	AVERAGE	55%	151/69
6.5	SLIGHT ABOVE	297/135		5.5	SLIGHT BELOW	52%	154/70
7	ABOVE	319/145		5	BELOW	49%	156/71
7.5	WAY ABOVE	341/155		4.5	WAY BELOW	46%	157/72

ABOVE AVERAGE NA/CNS POTENTIAL (74%)

MU/FIBER TYPE ENDURANCE POINT VALUE BASED ON QUANTITY				MU/FIBER TYPE STRENGTH POINT VALUE BASED ON QUANTITY		
	1	2A	2X		1	2A	2X
BELOW AVERAGE	1	1.5	2	BELOW AVERAGE	3	2	2.5
AVERAGE	2	3	1	AVERAGE	2	3	4
ABOVE AVERAGE	3	4.5	0	ABOVE AVERAGE	1	4	5.5

ESTIMATED 1-RM RESISTANCE FROM COMBINED STRENGTH POINTS (2A + 2X) AND ESTIMATED 35-RM RESISTANCE USED FROM COMBINED ENDURANCE POINTS (1 + 2A)

35-RM

STRENGTH POINTS	STRENGTH CATEGORY	1-RM (lbs./kgs.)		ENDURANCE POINTS	ENDURANCE CATEGORY	% used for 35-RM	35-RM (lbs./kgs.)
5.5	WAY BELOW	239/108		6.5	WAY ABOVE	61%	146/66
6	BELOW	264/120		6	ABOVE	58%	153/70
6.5	SLIGHT BELOW	289/131		5.5	SLIGHT ABOVE	55%	159/72
7	AVERAGE	314/143		5	AVERAGE	52%	163/74
7.5	SLIGHT ABOVE	339/154		4.5	SLIGHT BELOW	49%	166/75
8	ABOVE	364/166		4	BELOW	46%	167/76
8.5	WAY ABOVE	389/177		3.5	WAY BELOW	43%	167/76

BELOW AVERAGE NA/CNS POTENTIAL (66%)

MU/FIBER TYPE ENDURANCE POINT VALUE BASED ON QUANTITY				MU/FIBER TYPE STRENGTH POINT VALUE BASED ON QUANTITY			
	1	2A	2X		1	2A	2X
BELOW AVERAGE	2	2.5	3	BELOW AVERAGE	2	1	1.5
AVERAGE	3	4	2	AVERAGE	1	2	3
ABOVE AVERAGE	4	5.5	1	ABOVE AVERAGE	0	3	4.5

ESTIMATED 1-RM RESISTANCE FROM COMBINED STRENGTH POINTS
(2A + 2X) AND ESTIMATED 35-RM RESISTANCE USED FROM
COMBINED ENDURANCE POINTS (1 + 2A)

35-RM

STRENGTH POINTS	STRENGTH CATEGORY	1-RM (lbs./kgs.)		ENDURANCE POINTS	ENDURANCE CATEGORY	% used for 35-RM	35-RM (lbs./kgs.)
3.5	WAY BELOW	179/82		8.5	WAY ABOVE	67%	120/55
4	BELOW	198/90		8	ABOVE	64%	127/58
4.5	SLIGHT BELOW	217/99		7.5	SLIGHT ABOVE	61%	132/60
5	AVERAGE	236/107		7	AVERAGE	58%	137/62
5.5	SLIGHT ABOVE	255/116		6.5	SLIGHT BELOW	55%	140/64
6	ABOVE	274/124		6	BELOW	52%	142/65
6.5	WAY ABOVE	293/133		5.5	WAY BELOW	49%	143/65

1-RM U.O.F.

Section 1

TOT	70% @ MAX	NEED FOR THE 1-RM	END OF REP	REC. & FAT	REC. & NOT FAT.	RES. POOL
750	525	525	Start	0	525	750
750		525	1	0	525	750
750			2	0	525	750

Section 2A

TOT	70% @ MAX	NEED FOR THE 1-RM	END OF REP	REC. & FAT	REC. & NOT FAT.	RES. POOL
976	684	684	Start	0	684	976
976		684	1	0	684	976
976			2	0	684	976

Section 2X

TOT	70% @ MAX	NEED FOR THE 1-RM	END OF REP	REC. & FAT	REC. & NOT FAT	RES. POOL
786	550	550	Start	0	550	786
786		550	1	(276)	275	510
510			2	(276)	510	510

TOTALS

COMBINED TOTAL U.O.F. OF ALL NEEDED THE FOR 1-RM (100% of 70% at max effort)	TOTAL U.O.F. AVAILABLE FOR A 2nd REP	REASON FOR THE INABILITY TO COMPLETE A 2nd REP
1,759		
	2,236	FATIGUED (276) TYPE 2X
Recruitable @ 70% 510	1,719	

10-RM U.O.F.

Section 1

TOT	70% @ MAX	NEED FOR EACH REP	END OF REP	REC. & FAT	REC. & NOT FAT.	RES. POOL
750	525	525	Start	0	525	750
750			1	0	525	750
750			2	0	525	750
750			3	0	525	750
750			4	0	525	750
750			5	0	525	750
750			6	0	525	750
750			7	0	525	750
750			8	0	525	750
750			9	0	525	750
750			10	0	525	750
750			11	0		

Section 2A

TOT	70% @ MAX	NEED FOR EACH REP	END OF REP	REC. & FAT	REC. & NOT FAT	RES. POOL
976	684	684	Start	0	684	976
976			1	0	684	976
			2	0	684	976
			3	14	670	962
			4	(42)28	656	934
			5	(82)40	644	894
			6	(138)56	628	838
			7	(248)110	574	728
			8	(398)150	534	578
			9	(573)175	403	403
			10	(773)200	203	203
203			11	(773)	203	

Section 2X

TOT	70% @ MAX	NEED FOR EACH REP	END OF REP	REC. & FAT	REC. & NOT FAT	RES. POOL
786	550	126	Start	0	126	786
			1	5	121	781
			2	(14)9	117	772
			3	(28)14	112	758
			4	(48)20	106	738
			5	(75)27	99	711
			6	(110)35	91	676
			7	(154)44	82	632
			8	(208)54	72	578
			9	(314)106	126	472
			10	(531)217	190	255
255			11	(531)	255	255

TOTALS

COMBINED TOTAL U.O.F. OF ALL NEEDED FOR EACH REP OF THE 10-RM	TOTAL U.O.F. AVAILABLE FOR AN 11th REP	REASON FOR THE INABILITY TO COMPLETE AN 11th REP
1,335		
	1,208	FATIGUED: (773) TYPE 2A
Recruitable @ 70%	983	(531) TYPE 2X

35-RM U.O.F.

1

TOT. = 750 | 70% @ MAX = 525 | NEED FOR EACH REP = 525

END OF REP	REC. & FAT.	REC. & NOT FAT.	RES. POOL
Start	0	525	750
1	0	525	750
3	0	525	750
5	0	525	750
7	0	525	750
9	0	525	750
11	0	525	750
13	0	525	750
15	0	525	750
17	0	525	750
19	0	525	750
21	0	525	750
23	0	525	750
25	0	525	750
27	0	525	750
29	0	525	750
31	0	525	750
33	0	525	750
35	0	525	750
36	0	525	750

TOT. (bottom) = 750

2A

TOT. = 976 | 70% @ MAX = 525 | NEED FOR EACH REP = 488

END OF REP	REC. & FAT.	REC. & NOT FAT.	RES. POOL	TOT.
Start	0	488	976	706
1	0	488	976	
3	0	488	976	
5	0	488	976	
7	0	488	976	
9	0	488	976	
11	16	472	960	
13	(42)26	462	934	
15	(79)37	451	897	
17	(128)49	439	848	
19	(190)62	426	786	
21	(268)78	410	708	
23	(363)95	393	613	
25	(480)117	371	496	
27	(611)131	357	365	
29	(774)163	202	202	
31	(976)202	202	0	
33	0	0	0	
35	0	0	0	
36	(976)	0	0	460

TOT. (bottom) = 0

2X

TOT. = 706 | 70% @ MAX = 550 | NEED FOR EACH REP = 0

END OF REP	REC. & FAT.	REC. & NOT FAT.	RES. POOL
Start	0	0	786
1	0	0	786
3	0	0	786
5	0	0	786
7	0	0	786
9	0	0	786
11	0	0	786
13	0	0	786
15	0	0	786
17	0	0	786
19	0	0	786
21	0	0	786
23	0	0	786
25	0	0	786
27	0	0	786
29	31	92	755
31	(93)62	224	693
33	(190)97	391	596
35	(326)136	324	460
36	(326)	324	460

TOTALS

	COMBINED TOTAL U.O.F. OF ALL NEEDED FOR EACH REP OF THE 35-RM	TOTAL U.O.F. AVAILABLE FOR A 36th REP	REASON FOR THE INABILITY TO COMPLETE A 36th REP
	1,013	1,210	FATIGUED: (976) TYPE 2A
		985 (Recruitable @ 70%)	(326) TYPE 2X

AVERAGE CNS POTENTIAL + COMBINED ALL MU/FIBER QUANTITY POINT VALUES AND RESULTANT STRENGTH AND ENDURANCE POTENTIAL

STRENGTH POTENTIAL

POINTS	WAY BELOW			BELOW			SLIGHT BELOW			AVERAGE			SLIGHT ABOVE			ABOVE			WAY ABOVE		
5															5						5
4.5																					
4																					
3.5						3.5		3.5				3.5					3.5	3.5			
3																					
2.5		2.5									2.5					2.5			2.5	2.5	
2			2						2												
1.5					1.5		1.5			1.5			1.5	1.5							
1																					
0.5	0.5			0.5																	
	AA	A	BA	AA	BA	A	A	AA	BA	A	A	A	A	BA	AA	BA	AA	A	BA	A	AA
	1	2A	2X	1	2A	2X	1	2A	2X	1	2A	2X	1	2A	2X	1	2A	2X	1	2A	2X
TOTAL	**5**			**5.5**			**7**			**7.5**			**8**			**9.5**			**10**		

ENDURANCE POTENTIAL

POINTS	WAY BELOW			BELOW			SLIGHT BELOW			AVERAGE			SLIGHT ABOVE			ABOVE			WAY ABOVE		
5													5							5	
4.5																					
4																					
3.5					3.5		3.5				3.5					3.5	3.5				
3										3											
2.5	2.5																	2.5	2.5		2.5
2		2						2													
1.5				1.5					1.5			1.5	1.5		1.5						
1																					
0.5			0.5			0.5															
	A	BA	AA	BA	A	AA	AA	BA	A	A	A	A	BA	AA	A	AA	A	BA	A	AA	BA
	1	2A	2X	1	2A	2X	1	2A	2X	1	2A	2X	1	2A	2X	1	2A	2X	1	2A	2X
TOTAL	**5**			**5.5**			**7**			**7.5**			**8**			**9.5**			**10**		

ABOVE AVE. CNS POTENTIAL + COMBINED ALL MU/FIBER QUANTITY POINT VALUES AND RESULTANT STRENGTH AND ENDURANCE POTENTIAL

STRENGTH POTENTIAL

POINTS	WAY BELOW			BELOW			SLIGHT BELOW			AVERAGE			SLIGHT ABOVE			ABOVE			WAY ABOVE		
5.5															5.5						5.5
5																					
4.5																					
4			4				4					4					4	4			
3.5																					
3		3									3					3			3	3	
2.5			2.5						2.5												
2					2		2			2			2	2							
1.5																					
1	1			1																	
0.5																					
	AA	A	BA	AA	BA	A	A	AA	BA	A	A	A	A	BA	AA	BA	AA	A	BA	A	AA
	1	2A	2X	1	2A	2X	1	2A	2X	1	2A	2X	1	2A	2X	1	2A	2X	1	2A	2X
TOTAL	**6.5**			**7**			**8.5**			**9**			**9.5**			**11**			**11.5**		

ENDURANCE POTENTIAL

POINTS	WAY BELOW			BELOW			SLIGHT BELOW			AVERAGE			SLIGHT ABOVE			ABOVE			WAY ABOVE		
5.5																					
5																					
4.5														4.5						4.5	
4																					
3.5																					
3					3		3				3					3	3				
2.5																					
2	2									2								2	2		2
1.5		1.5						1.5													
1				1					1			1	1		1						
0.5			0			0															
	A	BA	AA	BA	A	AA	AA	BA	A	A	A	A	BA	AA	A	AA	A	BA	A	AA	BA
	1	2A	2X	1	2A	2X	1	2A	2X	1	2A	2X	1	2A	2X	1	2A	2X	1	2A	2X
TOTAL	**3.5**			**4**			**5.5**			**6**			**6.5**			**8**			**8.5**		

BELOW AVE. CNS POTENTIAL + COMBINED ALL MU/FIBER QUANTITY POINT VALUES AND RESULTANT STRENGTH AND ENDURANCE POTENTIALS

STRENGTH POTENTIAL

POINTS	WAY BELOW			BELOW			SLIGHT BELOW			AVERAGE			SLIGHT ABOVE			ABOVE			WAY ABOVE		
5.5																					
5																					
4.5															4.5						4.5
4																					
3.5																					
3						3	3					3					3	3			
2.5																					
2	2										2					2			2	2	
1.5			1.5						1.5												
1					1		1			1			1	1							
0.5	0			0																	
	AA	A	BA	AA	BA	A	A	AA	BA	A	A	A	A	BA	AA	BA	AA	A	BA	A	AA
	1	2A	2X	1	2A	2X	1	2A	2X	1	2A	2X	1	2A	2X	1	2A	2X	1	2A	2X
TOTAL	3.5			4			5.5			6			6.5			8			8.5		

ENDURANCE POTENTIAL

POINTS	WAY BELOW			BELOW			SLIGHT BELOW			AVERAGE			SLIGHT ABOVE			ABOVE			WAY ABOVE		
5.5														5.5						5.5	
5																					
4.5																					
4					4		4				4					4	4				
3.5																					
3	3									3								3	3		3
2.5		2.5						2.5													
2				2					2			2	2		2						
1.5																					
1			1			1															
0.5																					
	A	BA	AA	BA	A	AA	AA	BA	A	A	A	A	BA	AA	A	AA	A	BA	A	AA	BA
	1	2A	2X	1	2A	2X	1	2A	2X	1	2A	2X	1	2A	2X	1	2A	2X	1	2A	2X
TOTAL	6.5			7			8.5			9			9.5			11			11.5		

REFERENCES

CITED

1. Stefano S. and C. Reggiani, "Fiber Types in Mammalian Skeletal Muscle," Physiol Rev, 91: 1447 – 1531, 2001. doi: 10.1152/physrev.0031.2020.

2. Gandevia, S.C., "Spinal and supraspinal factors in human muscle fatigue," Physiol Rev, 2001: 81:1725–89.

3. Bottinelli R., Pellegrino M.A., Canepari M., Rossi R., and C. Reggiani, "Specific contributions of various muscle fibre types to human muscle performance: an in vitro study." J Electromyogr Kinesio, 1999 Apr: 9(2):87-95.

4. http://assets.cambridge.org/97805218/76292/excerpt/9780521876292_excerpt.pdf, accessed January 3, 2020.

5. https://nba.uth.tmc.edu/neuroscience/m/s3/chapter01.html, accessed November 20, 2019.

6. https://opentextbc.ca/anatomyandphysiology/chapter/10-4-nervous-system-control-of-muscle-tension/, accessed February 21, 2020.

7. https://emedicine.medscape.com/article/1141359-overview, accessed August 12, 2020.

8. https://www.scientistcindy.com/muscles-and-reflexes-lab.html, accessed May 15, 2020.

9. Neuroscience, 2nd. Ed. Purves. D, Augustine. G.J., Fitzpatrick, D., et al., editors. Neuroscience, 2nd ed., Sunderland (MA): Sinauer Associates: 2001.

10. https://en.wikipedia.org/wiki/File:Muscle_Force_Velocity_relationship.png, accessed May 21, 2020.

11. St Clair-Gibson, A. and T. D. Noakes, "Evidence for complex system integration and dynamic neural regulation of skeletal muscle recruitment during exercise in humans." Br J Sports Med, 2004: 38:797–806. doi: 10.1136/bjsm.2003.009852

12. Yue G.H., Ranganathan V.K., Siemionow V., et al, "Evidence of inability to fully activate human limb muscle," Muscle Nerve, 2000, 23:376–84.

13. Adams, G.R., R.T. Harris, D. Woodard, and G.A. Dudley, "Mapping of electrical muscle stimulation using MRI," J Appl Physiol 1985, Feb. 74(2):532-537.

14. Enoka R.M., "Eccentric contractions require unique activation strategies by the nervous system." J Appl Physiol, 1996: 81:2339–46.

15. *https://www.medium.com/@SandCResearch/what-determines-mechanical-tension-during-strength-training-acdf31b93e18, accessed August 11, 2020.*

16. *https://medium.com/@SandCResearch/do-eccentric-and-concentric-training-produce-different-types-of-muscle-growth-ec66197b0f5c, accessed August 11, 2020.*

17. *http://www.sci.sdsu.edu/movies/actin_myosin_gif.html, accessed January 7, 2020.*

18. *https://medium.com/@SandCResearch/why-does-central-nervous-system-cns-fatigue-happen-during-strength-training-e0af3f5e4989, accessed May 1, 2020.*

19. *Kirkendall, D.T., "Mechanism of Peripheral Fatigue,"* Med Sci Sports Exerc. *1990 Aug: 22(4):444-9.*

20. *https://www.health.harvard.edu/blog/how-much-protein-do-you-need-every-day-201506188096, accessed June 4, 2020.*

21. *https://medium.com/the-get-fit-gang/stimulating-reps-the-ultimate-guide-to-maximizing-muscle-growth-21c25a7593db, accessed September 2, 2020.*

22. *https://journals.physiology.org/doi/full/10.1152/classicessays.00025.2005, accessed July 15, 2020.*

OTHER

Adams G.R., Harris R.T., Woodard D., et al. "Mapping of electrical activity using MRI." J Appl Physiol, *2000: 74:532–7.*

Anosue K., M. Yoshida, K. Akazawa, and K. Fujii, "The Number of Active Motor Units and Their Firing Rates in Voluntary Contraction of Human Brachialis Muscle." Japanese Journal of Physiology, *1979: 29, 427-443.*

Bellemare F., Woods J.J., Johansson R.S., et al." Motor unit discharge rates in maximal voluntary contractions of three human muscles." J Neurophysiol, *1983: 50:1380–92.*

Botterman, B., Binder, M., and D. Stuart, "Functional Anatomy of the Association between Motor Units and Muscle Receptors," Amer Zool., *1978: 18:135-152.*

Cormie, P., McGuigan, M.R. and R.U. & Newton, "Developing Maximal Neuromuscular Power." Sports Med 41, *17–38 (2011). https://doi.org/10.2165/11537690-000000000-00000, accessed May 7, 2020.*

Enoka R.M. "Morphological features and activation patterns of motor units." J Clin Neurophysiol, *1995: 12:538–58.*

Favero T.G., Zable A.C., Colter D., et al. "Lactate inhibits Ca2+-activated Ca2+channel activity from skeletal muscle sarcoplasmic reticulum." J Appl Physiol, *1997: 82:447–52.*

Francini, F., Bencini, C. and R. Squecco, "Activation of L-type calcium channel in twitch skeletal muscle fibres of the frog," Journal of Physiology, *1996: 494.1, pp. 121-140.*

Guyton, A.C., Medical Physiology. *1991: 8th ed. Philadelphia: W.B. Saunders.*

Ikai M. and A.H. Steinhaus, "Some factors modifying the expression of human strength." J Appl Physiol, *1961: 16:157–63.*

Kay D., St. Clair-Gibson A., Mitchell M.J., et al. "Different neuromuscular recruitment patterns during eccentric, concentric and isometric contractions." J Electromyogr Kinesiol, *2000: 10:425–31.*

Kukulka C.G. and P. Clamann, "Comparison of the recruitment and discharge properties of motor units in human brachial biceps and adductor pollicis during isometric contraction." Brain Res, *1981: 219:45–55.*

St Clair Gibson A., Lambert M.I., and T.D. Noakes, "Neural control of force output during maximal and submaximal exercise." Sports Med, *2001: 31:637–50.*

Talbot, J. and L. Maves, "Skeletal muscle fiber type: using insights from muscle developmental biology to dissect targets for susceptibility and resistance to muscle disease," First published: 19 May, 2016, https://doi.org/10.1002/wdev.230, accessed January 23, 2020.

Tesch P.A., Dudley G.A., Duvoisin M.R., et al. "Force and EMG signal patterns during repeated bouts of concentric or eccentric muscle actions." Acta Physiol Scand, *1990: 138:263–71.*

http://assets.cambridge.org/97805218/76292/excerpt/9780521876292_excerpt.pdf, accessed March 7, 2020.

http://fig.cox.miami.edu/~cmallery/150/neuro/muscle.htm, accessed February 21, 2020.

http://perspectivesinmedicine.cshlp.org/content/7/10/a029702.short, accessed February 21, 2020.

https://bmcmusculoskeletdisord.biomedcentral.com/articles/10.1186/1471-2474-13-218, accessed May 5, 2020.

https://meat.tamu.edu/ansc-307-honors/muscle-contraction/, accessed February 21, 2020.

https://media.lanecc.edu/users/howardc/PTA101/101FoundationsofEstim/ 101FoundationsofEstim3.html, accessed January 24, 2020.

https://musculoskeletalkey.com/muscle-anatomy-physiology-and-biochemistry, accessed April 5, 2020.

https://opentextbc.ca/anatomyandphysiology/chapter/10-4-nervous-system-control-of-muscle-tension/, accessed January 4, 2020.

https://ouhsc.edu/bserdac/dthompso/web/namics/mu.htm, accessed April 8, 2020.

https://www.academia.edu/32630157/ Neuromuscular_Rehabilitation_in_Manual_and_Physical_Therapy_Principles_to_Practice, accessed December 4, 2019.

https://www.ncbi.nlm.nih.gov/pmc/articles/PMC5180455/, accessed May 30, 2020.

https://www.ptdirect.com/training-design/anatomy-and-physiology/skeletal-muscle-2013-anatomy-and-fiber-types, accessed February 23, 2020.

https://www.youtube.com/watch?v=MLSxhTGkkPc, accessed March 18, 2020.

ABOUT THE AUTHOR

I am currently an Exercise Physiologist with the St. Louis Metropolitan Police Department. I also train clients through Pinnacle Personal and Performance Training in Chesterfield, MO. For 23 years I was in the collegiate strength and conditioning profession, serving as the Head Coach for Strength and Conditioning at Saint Louis University (2004-2008), the University of Illinois at Chicago (2001-2004), Southeast Missouri State University (1991-2001) and the University of Florida (1988-1990). I got my start in the strength and conditioning field as an Assistant Strength Coach at Florida in 1984 where I was also a weight training instructor for the Department of Physical Education from 1985 to 1988.

In 2006, I was named Master Strength and Conditioning Coach by the Collegiate Strength and Conditioning Coaches Association for my years of service in the field. In 1999, I was named NSCA Ohio Valley Conference Strength and Conditioning Professional of the year. In 2001, I received an honorary certification from the International Association of Resistance Trainers (I.A.R.T.).

I possess C.S.C.S. and S.C.C.C. certifications with the National Strength and Conditioning Association and Collegiate Strength and Conditioning Coaches Association, respectively. Additionally, I am certified by the Illinois Law Enforcement Training and Standards Board in basic instructor development and as a Specialist Instructor by the Missouri Department of Public Safety. In 2012, I became certified by the IBNFC as a Certified Nutrition Coach.

I have also worked with athletes at the Olympic and professional levels, presented at various clinics/seminars, and worked several athletic-related camps. I am a strong advocate of safe, practical, and time-efficient training and have published a collection of periodical articles, book chapters, complete books, and user-friendly downloads promoting such. My six solo projects, *The Interval Training Manual, The Ultimate*

Interval and Circuit Training Manual, The Strength Training Workout Encyclopedia, 100 Old School Strength Training Workouts, 25 Kick-Butt Workouts, and *85 Workouts of the Week* are one-of-a-kind references for anyone seeking guidelines to improve strength, fitness and lose body fat. I also wrote over 190 articles for the popular web site breakingmuscle.com where I also designed several Mature Athlete workout training programs.

I received a Bachelor's Degree from the University of Iowa in 1981 (It's Great to be a Hawkeye!) and a Master's Degree in Physical Education from Western Illinois University in 1984. I was a member of the Track and Field team at Iowa and served as a Graduate Assistant Track and Field Coach while at Western Illinois.